Rapid Adult Nursing

Rapid Adult Nursing

Andrée le May
Professor Emerita of Nursing
School of Health Sciences
University of Southampton

WILEY Blackwell

This edition first published 2017 © 2017 by John Wiley and Sons, Ltd

Registered Office
John Wiley & Sons, Ltd, The Atrium, Southern Gate, Chichester, West Sussex, PO19 8SQ, UK

Editorial Offices
9600 Garsington Road, Oxford, OX4 2DQ, UK
The Atrium, Southern Gate, Chichester, West Sussex, PO19 8SQ, UK
111 River Street, Hoboken, NJ 07030-5774, USA

For details of our global editorial offices, for customer services and for information about how to apply for permission to reuse the copyright material in this book please see our website at www.wiley.com/wiley-blackwell

The right of the author to be identified as the author of this work has been asserted in accordance with the UK Copyright, Designs and Patents Act 1988.

Library of Congress Cataloging-in-Publication Data

Names: Le May, Andrée, author.
Title: Rapid adult nursing / Andrée le May.
Description: Chichester, West Sussex ; Hoboken, NJ : John Wiley & Sons, Inc., 2017. | Includes bibliographical references and index.
Identifiers: LCCN 2016020348 | ISBN 9781119117117 (pbk.) | ISBN 9781119117124 (Adobe PDF) | ISBN 9781119117131 (epub)
Subjects: | MESH: Nursing | Nursing Care—methods | Adult | Handbooks
Classification: LCC RT51 | NLM WY 49 | DDC 610.73–dc23
LC record available at https://lccn.loc.gov/2016020348

A catalogue record for this book is available from the British Library.

Wiley also publishes its books in a variety of electronic formats. Some content that appears in print may not be available in electronic books.

Cover image: © sturti/iStock

Set in 7.5/9.5pt Frutiger by SPi Global, Pondicherry, India
Printed and bound in Malaysia by Vivar Printing Sdn Bhd
1   2017

Contents

Introduction

This book brings together up-to-date evidence and essential knowledge from various sources in an easy-to-follow, 'quick' introductory or revision text for student nurses.

It is designed to give you rapid access to key information. It is not designed to give you comprehensive information – you will need to read around the subject areas highlighted in this book to get that.

The first section provides information related to the essential components of excellent nursing, highlighting the skills that all students need to develop from the outset of their studies. The second section focuses on common conditions that you are likely to encounter.

Acknowledgements

The author is grateful to the following authors on whose works she drew in compiling this book.

Brooker C and Nicol M (2011) (Eds) Alexander's Nursing Practice. Edinburgh, Churchill Livingstone Elsevier.

Davey P (2010) (Ed.) Medicine at a Glance. Oxford, Wiley Blackwell.

Dougherty L and Lister S (2011) (Eds) The Royal Marsden Hospital Manual of Clinical Nursing Procedures. Student Edition. Oxford, Wiley Blackwell.

Gabbay J and le May A (2011) Practice-Based Evidence for Healthcare: Clinical Mindlines. Abingdon, Routledge.

Grace P and Borley N (2009) (Eds) Surgery at a Glance. Oxford, Wiley Blackwell.

le May A (2015) Adult Nursing at a Glance. Oxford, Wiley Blackwell.

le May A and Holmes S (2012) Introduction to Nursing Research: Developing Research Awareness. London, Hodder Arnold.

Macintosh M and Moore T (2011) (Eds) Caring for the Seriously Ill Patient. London, Hodder Arnold.

O'Brien L (2012) (Ed.) District Nursing Manual of Clinical Procedures. Oxford, Wiley Blackwell.

Peate I and Nair M (2011) (Eds) Fundamentals of Anatomy and Physiology for Student Nurses. Oxford, Wiley Blackwell.

Part 1 Fundamentals of Nursing Care

Rapid Adult Nursing, First Edition. Andrée le May.
© 2017 John Wiley & Sons, Ltd. Published 2017 by John Wiley & Sons, Ltd.

Adult nursing
Definition
Adult nursing comprises the skilled, dignified care of adults. It focuses on acute and chronic physical conditions rather than mental illness. Adults are nursed in a variety of settings – the community, hospitals and longer-term care settings.

Excellent care for adults through their lifespan is about what nurses do, and how nurses do it, in partnership with patients, their families and carers, as well as in collaboration with other members of the multi-disciplinary health and social care team.

Fundamental to excellent nursing is the merging of technically competent care with the maintenance and/or enhancement of the patient's (and their family's and carer's) dignity.

Care that is technically competent but does not promote the patient's dignity is inadequate; care that promotes dignity but is not technically competent is also inadequate. Excellent nursing is therefore underpinned by the following:

- Safeguarding dignity.
- Skilled, appropriate communication.
- Accurate assessment and monitoring.
- Tailored symptom control and management.
- Attentive risk assessment and management.
- Tailored health education and promotion.
- Thorough discharge planning.
- Evaluation of the outcomes of care and care processes.
- Use of the best evidence from research, theory, audit and service/practice development.

Nurses are accountable for the care they provide and must practise within the legal and ethical frameworks laid down by their professional and regulatory bodies.

Assessment and monitoring
Definition
Assessment is the systematic collection of key information to inform care. Monitoring is the regular updating of this information. Assessment and monitoring are iterative processes.

Accurate assessment and ongoing monitoring of a patient's physical and mental health are critical to the provision of effective, safe and timely care and the plotting of progress/ deterioration. Assessment and monitoring of the patient's relatives' responses to the illness/condition and its consequences also need to be conducted. All nurses, regardless of the healthcare setting in which they work, undertake various types of assessment and monitoring.

Skilled assessment is linked to the ability to prioritise care that needs to be done urgently (e.g. through using early-warning scales) and care that can wait.

Successful assessment and monitoring involve nurses merging hard data (e.g. from measurement equipment and assessment scales) with soft data (e.g. from talking, watching and listening to patients, their families and their healthcare team members) to form a complete picture of the patient's condition and their response(s) to it and to nursing care and treatments.

Assessments can range from the comprehensive (e.g. covering physical, psychological, social, emotional, spiritual and cultural dimensions) to the specific (e.g. taking a temperature or monitoring wound healing).

Making a comprehensive nursing assessment should be done in partnership with the patient and their family/carers and it underpins the delivery of care. All nursing assessments should inform and be informed by those made by other health and social care workers.

The specific assessment and monitoring of elements of a patient's health can help in the early detection of general health problems (e.g. hypertension); in establishing the effectiveness of treatments (e.g. in type 1 diabetes); in determining the progression of an acute illness (e.g. an infection) or a long-term condition (e.g. multiple sclerosis), the impact of one type of illness on another (e.g. an acute respiratory infection on asthma) and the generation of one illness because of another (e.g. depression resulting from chronic obstructive pulmonary disease).

Accurate baseline assessments are essential if improvement or deterioration of a patient's health is to be identified swiftly and managed appropriately through ongoing monitoring.

The results of assessment and monitoring need to be accurately recorded in a patient's care plan or notes.

Initial assessments and deviations from the expected course of a patient's condition need to be effectively communicated to relevant healthcare team members. Using a structured approach to communicating your assessment and planning (e.g. SBAR: Situation, Background, Assessment and Recommendation) can be useful in effectively explaining requirements to patients, their families and members of the multi-disciplinary team.

Following an initial nursing assessment, the majority of ongoing monitoring is likely to focus on four key areas:

• The patient's physical health and present condition set against the treatment plan.
• The patient's mental health and present condition set against the treatment plan.
• Any special requirements the patient has.
• The patient's and the carer's requirements for social support.

Audit
Definition
Audit is a cyclical process of measuring care against agreed criteria (or standards), deciding whether alterations need to be made to care, making changes, and measuring again to see whether the change has been effective. Audits are used to provide information that can help inform best practice and should be carried out regularly.

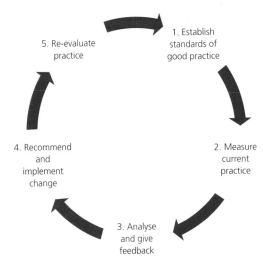

1. Establish standards of good practice
2. Measure current practice
3. Analyse and give feedback
4. Recommend and implement change
5. Re-evaluate practice

Figure 1 The clinical audit cycle.

Audit can be done either at a national or at a local level.

Copeland (2005, p. 16) provided the following criteria to help practitioners develop a good local audit:

1. Should be part of a structured programme.
2. Topics chosen should in the main be high risk; high volume or high cost or reflect National Clinical Audits, NSFs (National Service Frameworks) or NICE [National Institute for Health and Care Excellence] guidance.
3. Service users should be part of the clinical audit process.
4. Should be multidisciplinary in nature.
5. Clinical audit should include assessment of process and outcome of care.
6. Standards should be derived from good quality guidelines.
7. The sample size chosen should be adequate to produce credible results.
8. Managers should be actively involved in audit and in particular in the development of action plans from audit enquiry.
9. Action plans should address the local barriers to change and identify those responsible for service improvement.
10. Re-audit should be applied to ascertain whether improvements in care have been implemented as a result of clinical audit.
11. Systems, structures and specific mechanisms should be made available to monitor service improvements once the audit cycle has been completed.
12. Each audit should have a local lead.

Communication
Definition
Communication is the transfer of information between one person and another, and their reaction to it. Communication permeates everything that nurses do, and being able to communicate effectively with patients, their families/carers and colleagues is an essential feature of skilled nursing practice. Skilled communication enhances care.

Communication includes a variety of different verbal and non-verbal cues and skills. Verbal communication comprises speech and language – this includes the way we use words, tones and inflections; the way we phrase what we say; and the questions that we ask in order to communicate what we are thinking and feeling. Non-verbal communication involves many things: touch, facial expressions, eye contact and the way we look at each other, gestures, body movements, posture and body positions, our use of space, the clothes we wear and our appearance, and even the timing of communication. Non-verbal communication supports verbal communication, but it is a powerful way of communicating information on its own. Silence is also a powerful means of communication.

Written communications are important to convey information between members of the multi-disciplinary team and to help patients and their families/carers retain information about their illness and treatment.

Communication is influenced by many things, including culture, age, mood, emotion, uncertainty, stress, anxiety, knowledge and skills. When considering patients and their families, it is important to remember that the effectiveness of communication can be affected by age-related or disease-linked problems, such as hearing loss, sight loss or alterations, speech alterations, emotions, mood, memory changes and cognitive impairment. Nurses need to minimise these barriers and also to reduce organisational barriers such as lack of privacy, having insufficient time to clarify uncertainties or misunderstandings, and communicating complicated information in noisy environments that make talking and hearing difficult. Altered mental capacity may mean that a patient is unable to communicate their wishes, understand information given to them or use it in decision making.

When communicating within the multi-disciplinary team, it is also important to reduce barriers associated with busyness, stress and status. Using a structured approach to communication such as SBAR (i.e. giving details of the current Situation your patient is in, providing essential Background to this, giving your Assessment of what is happening and your Recommendation about what needs to happen next) is useful, especially in situations where urgent attention and clarity of information are needed.

Effective communication is about using the right verbal and non-verbal skills for the person (or people) involved in each interaction. Useful communication skills include:

- Establishing rapport.
- Active and empathic listening.
- Responding and being able to summarise information accurately.
- Not being afraid to keep quiet (or to speak out).
- Using questions to find out more (particularly open questions).
- Using reinforcement (e.g. 'go on', nodding) to encourage communication.
- Using story-telling to find out more or engage people in conversation as appropriate.
- Using touch appropriately, particularly expressive touch.
- Observing people's reactions and changing your communication style in response.
- Being non-judgemental and open.
- Showing respect and maintaining dignity through both actions and words.
- Remembering that the 'little things' (e.g. smiling and eye contact) are important.
- Evaluating how well your interactions with people go is important in either reinforcing effective skills or improving things for next time.

Continuing professional development
Definition

Continuing professional development (CPD) is about ensuring that your knowledge and skills are up to date and that you remain competent to practise throughout your career. CPD is something that every healthcare professional has to do.

CPD is sometimes described as continuing personal and professional development (CPPD), and this reflects the breadth of opportunities that can count as CPD.

The Nursing and Midwifery Council (NMC) requirements for CPD must be met every time you renew your registration. For nurses working in the UK, CPD may include regularly updating skills and knowledge, reflecting on practice and their day-to-day work and teaching/mentoring others. All of these involve continuous learning and development. Taking part in and implementing the learning gained from these activities enables nurses to give safe, up-to-date, highly skilled care.

CPD is not, for instance, just about going on courses and collecting certificates – it involves thinking about how you will use your learning to develop yourself as well as your care. This self-development can be structured by writing a personal development plan (PDP) and sharing it with your manager or mentor. A PDP helps you plan what you intend to learn or improve in the future. Clinical supervision also helps with your personal development.

All the CPD you do should be recorded in a portfolio. This will provide you with a useful record of what you have achieved, which will be helpful for constructing your curriculum vitae or for presentation to the NMC if it checks your CPD activities when you re-register/re-validate. Your portfolio should document what you have done, what you have learnt from it and how it has influenced your practice; it should make reference to your PDP.

CPD does not just have to be about developing clinical knowledge and skills. It is important to develop other skills as well in order to enhance the care that you provide. For example, you might choose to develop some managerial skills, delegation skills or leadership skills – all of these will make you a more competent practitioner.

All in all, CPD is about making you a more accomplished nurse.

Dignity
Definition

Dignity is often said to be hard to define. The available definitions tend to focus on either the professional view of dignity or the public's view. The challenge is to integrate them.

Professional definitions of dignity are frequently abstract and are inclined to focus on the behaviours, values and attitudes that professionals need to have. For example, 'Dignity is concerned with how people feel, think and behave in relation to the worth or value of themselves and others. To treat someone with dignity is to treat them as being of worth, in a way that is respectful of them as valued individuals' (RCN, 2008).

Public reports (e.g. Francis, 2013) and research (e.g. Cairns et al., 2013), however, suggest that patients and the public see dignity in more pragmatic terms, focusing on whether or not certain important aspects of daily living can be completed while relying on others for assistance. These include having privacy, being able to go to the toilet when needed, being able to wash after using the toilet, having food and drink that can be consumed when needed and when wanted, being helped with eating and drinking if necessary, being listened to and having opinions respected.

Integrating the professional and the public views of dignity is important to the provision of excellent care, so that patients and their family feel that they have experienced competent, individualised care that allows them to maintain their dignity. Dignity is maintained in the following ways.

What nurses do, for instance:

- Work with patients and their families/carers to identify and understand their individual needs and decide, with them, what care is required to meet these needs.
- Undertake such care in a timely and respectful manner.

How nurses do it, for instance:

- Treat each patient as an individual.
- Listen to and respect their views.
- Work in partnership with each patient and their family/carers.
- Offer choice wherever possible.
- Promote privacy.
- Ensure that people can voice satisfaction and dissatisfaction with care without fearing reprisal.

When nurses do it, for instance:

- Identify with patients (and their family/carers) mutually convenient times for care whenever possible.
- Ensure that medications, designed to fit the patient's needs rather than the treatment plan, are given on time (particularly night sedation).
- Question practice that they think is inappropriate.

Discharge planning

Definition

Discharge planning always occurs in partnership with the patient and their family/carers as well as with other members of the multi-disciplinary team. Planning a person's discharge from nursing care should start during their initial assessment, when care is being planned and agreed. For patients having surgery or any other planned procedure, discharge planning will have been discussed during their pre-assessment visit. In primary care, discharge from nursing care is usually negotiated between the patient, their family/carers and the nursing team/nurse.

In hospital wards, patients are often given an expected date of discharge (EDD) once their medical condition has been stabilised. Having an EDD helps all members of the multi-disciplinary team, the patient and their family/carers plan ahead.

Discharge planning is usually led by a senior member in the nursing team or the patient's key worker. A person's discharge from any care environment should be coordinated, efficiently undertaken and, where appropriate, ensure the smooth passage of a person's care from one service to another. Hospitals will have discharge policies to guide discharge planning. Some wards will have their own tailored policy.

Inadequate discharge planning can result in patients and their families/carers being unprepared for the realities of returning home from hospital or transferring to another care environment (e.g. a nursing or residential home), or in them receiving unsuitable care. Poor discharge planning may mean that patients have to stay in hospital longer or are re-admitted, or that they recover less well.

Discharge planning should take into account all the aspects of a comprehensive assessment (e.g. the physical, psychological, social, emotional, spiritual and cultural dimensions). For some people, it will also be necessary during this process to discuss economic and environmental factors, such as housing, benefits and return to work, alongside daily routines such as shopping and cooking.

Referral to members of the multi-disciplinary team for assessment should be made as soon as possible.

Some patients may decide to discharge themselves from hospital against medical advice and this needs to be reported appropriately and recorded.

Some people will have particular care needs following discharge from hospital or transfer between services. This group includes people who are elderly, who are dying, whose condition is unpredictable, who live alone, who require equipment with which they are not yet familiar, who are homeless or live in poor housing conditions, and those with learning difficulties or ongoing health problems.

Effective discharge is achieved when:

- The discharge plan is agreed in partnership with the patient, their family/carers and the multi-disciplinary team.
- The patient and family/carers are fully informed of the plan and help shape it.
- A named nurse/key worker is appointed to coordinate a patient's discharge from any healthcare service.
- All relevant documents are updated and information is transferred to all appropriate services in time to ensure that continuity of care is maintained.
- Relevant services are introduced into the care package at the right time to ensure continuity of care.
- Success is monitored.
- Deviations from the plan are identified and corrected.

Documentation
Definition
Clearly, succinctly and accurately recording care given, or to be given, is a vital part of communication within the healthcare team and between services. Accurate documentation promotes continuity of care.

Professional and statutory bodies lay down guidance for record keeping. Care and observations of a patient's condition are recorded through a variety of paper and/or electronic means, including:

- Patient records (e.g. including nursing assessments)
- Care plans
- Medication charts
- Observational charts (e.g. vital signs, fluid balance, Glasgow Coma Scale, pain scales)
- Printouts from monitors (e.g. ECGs [electrocardiograms])
- Risk assessment charts (e.g. early warning scores, pressure ulcer risk assessment)
- Letters/emails/text messages
- Photographs (e.g. of wounds)

Written information (either on paper or electronically) is an indispensable way of recording care and should be presented so that it can be understood by any reader. Information should be recorded clearly without using ambiguous terms or abbreviations. Where handwriting is used, it should be legible and in ink.

While record keeping is an essential part of care, all necessary steps should be taken not to allow it to drive patient care or to intrude excessively into the time devoted to patient contact.

Eating and drinking
Definition
Eating and drinking the right things are important in maintaining health and aiding recovery from illnesses, surgery or accidents. The body requires particular nutrients to stay healthy (proteins, fats, carbohydrates, vitamins, minerals and fluids). In ill health or following surgery, the body may require extra nutrients for repair. Imbalances of nutrients can alter the body's homeostasis.

Eating and drinking are social activities, and doing them alone may increase feelings of social isolation in some groups of people (e.g. older people eating by themselves in their rooms in residential or nursing homes).

Malnutrition is any imbalance between the person's nutritional needs and their diet. It can be assessed using the Malnutrition Universal Screening Tool (MUST).

Eating and drinking difficulties can occur for a variety of reasons, for example nausea and/or vomiting; a sore mouth or ill-fitting dentures; difficulty swallowing; difficulty using equipment such as cutlery following paralysis or as a result of severe dementia; anorexia; early satiety; allergies or intolerances; or particular diseases (e.g. diabetes).

Nurses, alongside dieticians, catering staff, occupational therapists, physiotherapists, speech and language therapists and healthcare assistants, have an important role to play in making sure that patients consume an appropriate diet. This is not merely about eating and drinking the right things, it is also about the functional ability to eat and drink (e.g. having sufficient dexterity to open food packaging, having dentures that fit and are in place, being able to reach drinks or meals that are left at the bedside, having the right adapted cutlery/plates/mats or being able to swallow).

Nurses need to assess whether a patient has consumed an appropriate amount of food and drink each day. This will involve finding out whether food is left uneaten, why this happened and making appropriate changes.

Nutrition screening will include:

- Asking about usual diet (food and drink).
- Asking about food preferences/allergies.
- Asking about normal food habits (e.g. Does the patient usually eat breakfast? Which meal is the largest during the day? Does the patient eat sandwiches for supper?).
- Discussing feeding difficulties (e.g. using special cutlery, ill-fitting dentures, sore mouth).
- Checking weight, height and Body Mass Index (BMI) on admission or more regularly.
- Checking BMI in primary care to determine the need for lifestyle changes in relation to weight gain or loss.
- Observing the patient (e.g. pallor, skin tone, under/overweight, oedema, mood).
- Noting results from blood tests (e.g. for anaemia).
- Evaluating nutritional intake (e.g. Are meals left unfinished? Is there a mismatch between fluid intake and output? Does the person feel hungry after eating?).

Some people will require nutritional support, for example oral supplements/sip feeds (high calories, high protein or high vitamin), or feeding using special preparations put directly into the gastro-intestinal tract via a naso-gastric (NG) tube or a percutaneous endoscopic gastrostomy (PEG), or intravenously using total parenteral nutrition (TPN).

Some people will have special dietary requirements. For instance, people with coeliac disease require a gluten-free diet, people with constipation may require a high-fibre diet, people with heart failure or cirrhosis of the liver may have a low-salt diet to help, alongside diuretics, control oedema.

Evaluation
Definition
Evaluation is about judging how effective nursing has been and is therefore closely linked to monitoring and assessment. Evaluation is used here to refer to an assessment of a completed episode of care, whereas monitoring is seen as a continuous evaluative exercise that is iterated with assessment.

At a broad level, evaluation centres on determining whether a patient's condition has improved, remained stable or deteriorated. At a more specific level, the achievement (or not) of each patient-centred goal set during the assessment process should be evaluated. Each goal should have an accompanying measurable outcome (e.g. the patient will walk for 20 minutes each day) that can be evaluated. Understanding why a patient does not reach goals is important to planning future care, both for the patient and for others. Understanding what has helped a patient to reach goals, but was not part of the care plan, is also useful.

A patient's and their family's/carer's satisfaction with care can also be evaluated and this can be done by asking them or by using a short satisfaction survey.

The results of individual patient evaluations should be recorded in the care plan or nursing notes and communicated to others in the multi-disciplinary team as required. Individual evaluations can be collated in audits to get a broader view of how successful care has been.

Discussing evaluations within the nursing team or the multi-disciplinary team can help to improve care or celebrate successful care, and also help to identify areas for audit.

Evaluations should be done against agreed outcomes, which should be 'SMART':

- Specific
- Measurable
- Achievable
- Realistic
- Timely

Evidence-based practice
Definition

Evidence-based practice is usually defined as 'the application of valid, relevant research-based information in nurse decision making' (Cullum et al., 2008, p. 2). While applying valid and relevant research to practice is essential, it is also important to remember that rigorous and relevant research may not always be available to base practice on. In this case, practitioners need to consider what other sorts of evidence could be used to support effective and efficient care. Other sources of evidence might include:

- Evidence from structured evaluations of practice (audit or other analyses of safety records, complaints etc.).
- Evidence from theory that is not grounded in research.
- Evidence from your experiences (professional and general).
- Evidence from your patients and/or their families and carers.
- Evidence passed on by role models/experts.
- Evidence from policy directives or guidelines.

Sometimes none of these is relevant and you have to search more widely for knowledge to help you to provide appropriate care. This might include searching for unpublished evidence in reports, research abstracts or conference proceedings using the internet or the media. Wherever the evidence comes from, it will require careful appraisal before it can be implemented. Attention needs to be paid to establishing the rigour of the evidence – research or otherwise. For research evidence this is primarily about reliability and validity and there are many crib sheets and tools that can help you do this (e.g. the series of CASP tools available at http://www.casp-uk.net/). For other sorts of evidence you should establish authenticity and robustness. To do this you might try to find out, for instance, the extent to which the evidence has been used elsewhere or evaluated before you use it.

Once you have decided that the evidence is suitable for use, it is important to establish its clinical relevance to the situation in which you intend to use it. Use these questions to help you do this (le May, 1999 and le May & Gabbay, 2010):

Is the evidence relevant clinically for the client?

1. What benefits will the implementation of this evidence have for patients/carers/staff?
2. What risks are associated with implementation/non-implementation?

Can the evidence be used by the organisation within which care is being given?

1. Are there enough resources for implementation?
2. What are the opportunities for and constraints to implementing this evidence?

Once you have established that the evidence can be trusted and is clinically relevant to your client, then you can use it in your practice and evaluate its effects and usefulness.

Fundamentals of nursing care
Definition
Excellent care is about what we do and how we do it.

Fundamental to excellent nursing is the merging of technically competent care with the maintenance and/or enhancement of the patient's (and their family's and carer's) dignity.

Care that is technically competent but does not promote the patient's dignity is inadequate; care that promotes dignity but is not technically competent is also inadequate. Excellent nursing is therefore underpinned by the following:

- Safeguarding dignity.
- Skilled, appropriate communication.
- Accurate assessment and monitoring.
- Tailored symptom control and management.
- Attentive risk assessment and management.
- Tailored health education and promotion.
- Thorough discharge planning.
- Evaluation of the outcomes of care and care processes.
- The use of the best evidence from research, theory, audit and service/practice development.

Health education and promotion
Definition
The World Health Organisation (WHO) defines health education as 'any combination of learning experiences designed to help individuals and communities improve their health, by increasing their knowledge and influencing their attitudes'.

Health promotion is defined by the WHO as 'the process of enabling people to increase control over, and to improve, their health. It moves beyond a focus on individual behaviour towards a wide range of social and environmental interventions.'

Increased knowledge and changed behaviour in individuals and communities/populations are the goals of health education and promotion. Behaviour change can occur as a result of a person changing what they do (e.g. stopping smoking), or by governments making laws that alter many people's behaviours (e.g. banning smoking in public places), or by communities exerting pressure to change behaviour (e.g. publicising the effects of passive smoking).

Educating people about their health and encouraging them to lead healthier lifestyles and to feel in control of their health and alterations to it are essential features of nursing.

All nurses, whatever their practice setting, will be involved in educating patients and their families/carers about health, and ways to improve their health or maintain a healthy lifestyle. These can range from education about medication to how to increase exercise and reduce weight. Some nurses, largely public health nurses and occupational health nurses, will take part in developing local and national policy on health improvements or creating healthy workplaces, hospitals and schools.

The basic principles of educating someone about health issues are:

• Work out what the person needs to know.
• Work out what the person does know.
• Work out the best way to fill the gap (if there is one), starting from where the person is.

Remember that when people are ill/uncomfortable/anxious their concentration level may be low, so it is important to be clear and concise in what you say and to use simple, easy-to-follow language. Make sure that you give information in small chunks and check out the person's understanding of what you said. It is useful to supplement oral information with written information. Always tell a person where to get advice if they forget what you say or something unexpected or unexplained happens, and if possible set up another time to check out what they know as a result of your intervention.

Infection prevention and control
Definition
Infection control and prevention are part of everyone's life. For example, we wash our hands after using the toilet or before we eat, and we stay at home when we are ill and likely to pass on infections to other people.

Nurses deliver care to people who may be infectious or vulnerable to cross-infection from other people, and so need to take extra precautions. Nurses protect people against infections in several ways. These include:

- Health education and promotion (e.g. teaching about infection control, encouraging vaccinations and immunisations).
- Preventing cross-infection between patients in hospital or in the community by vigilant hand washing (or the use of alcohol gel); the correct use of gloves, gowns and masks; the correct disposal of infected materials and sharps; and the use of isolation if appropriate (either to protect an immunocompromised person from developing infection or to stop other patients from coming into contact with someone whose illness is contagious).
- Preventing wound infections, bladder infections or intravenous infusion (IVI) site infections by using scrupulous aseptic techniques.
- Recognising infection so that treatment can be started as soon as possible (e.g. acting on changes in vital signs – elevated temperature, respirations or pulse; noticing heat, swelling, redness, pus or pain at the site of the infection; acting on reports of feelings of general malaise, confusion and specific condition-related responses, e.g. nausea, vomiting and diarrhoea in gastro-intestinal infections or frequency of micturition in urinary tract infections or cough with/without sputum in respiratory tract infections).
- Ensuring that anti-infective medications are taken as prescribed.
- Ensuring that the rules of basic hygiene are adhered to, for instance offering bed-bound patients hand-washing or hand-cleansing facilities after using a bedpan, bottle or commode, and before meals.

Leadership
Definition

Leadership is often described as being about our relationships with other people and the way we constructively influence them, and how we make things happen in teams, services and/or organisations. There are three key interacting elements in this influencing relationship within nursing: the leader, the people/person being influenced (sometimes known as followers, especially when we are thinking about teams of people) and the job/task being done. In nursing particularly, the job/task often involves other groups of people – either patients/service users and their families and carers or our health and social care colleagues. Leadership is largely about people and the way they communicate and behave.

Nurses are leaders in many situations – they lead episodes of care with patients and their friends and families; they lead teams of people providing care or those taking part in service development or improvement projects; they lead groups of students through mentorship and their peers through clinical supervision; and they lead health and social care organisations at various levels, from team leader to chief executive. Whatever the situation in which nurses are leading, the core element in that leadership process/relationship is ensuring that the most appropriate and effective care possible is given. Nurses often do that by influencing other people.

Good leaders are generally thought to have some or all of the following personal qualities and abilities: they are calm, enthusiastic, courageous and self-motivating; they have humility and integrity; they are seen to be tough but fair; and they possess and represent the qualities expected or required by the group of people they are leading. They use these qualities to help them to influence others, articulate their vision clearly, make and take decisions, work creatively and collaboratively, and be responsive and flexible. They motivate and encourage others to use their talents while being politically astute.

Leading people successfully requires nurses to be resourceful and adapt their leadership style and approach to suit the range of different situations (and people) that they encounter every day. Whoever or whatever it is that nurses are leading, their leadership needs to be clear, consistent and strong in order to ensure that dignified, high-quality care is delivered within a positive and supportive working environment.

Management
Definition

Management, just like leadership, is about working with and influencing people. Unlike leadership, the main purpose of management is to achieve the goals of the organisation. Management is therefore largely associated with specific, goal-oriented functions. Leaders do not generally have to achieve the same goal-oriented work as managers and so may be more able to be creative in what they do.

Planning, organising, motivating and controlling are the common functions of management (Rigolosi, 2013); although these functions can be described separately, they are often interlinked. *Planning* is about identifying problems, detailing long- and short-term goals, deciding on objectives and then working out how the goals and objectives are to be achieved. Goals and objectives need to be kept simple, meaningful, achievable and realistic; they also need to have a timescale attached to them (this is sometimes referred to as setting SMART goals/objectives). *Organising* is about getting together all the resources needed to achieve your goals – these resources include not only people with the right knowledge and skills, but also finance and equipment. *Motivating* other people to achieve the goals that are set is an important and sometimes challenging aspect of management. If people are not motivated they will not work effectively or efficiently, and this will have a negative impact on the organisation's effectiveness. Goal setting must therefore not only reflect the abilities of the people involved and available resources, but also the team and manager's motivation. *Controlling* does not mean controlling in terms of stopping people doing things or being manipulative; here controlling is about setting up ways to evaluate progress, either at the end of a job/project (summative evaluation) or at points during the job in order to act on this feedback (formative evaluation) to make the job go better. This ongoing, formative type of evaluation means that if necessary, plans can be adjusted as jobs/projects progress.

Managers need several particular skills to function well. These can be categorised as technical, human and conceptual skills. Sometimes technical skills are referred to as 'hard' skills and human skills as 'soft' skills. Technical skills are associated with using the appropriate knowledge, techniques and equipment to perform a task or achieve a goal (e.g. showing a junior member of the ward team how to set up an ECG or collating information using a particular software package). Human skills are about working with people and enabling them to contribute effectively to meeting goals. This involves understanding what motivates people and being able to communicate easily and clearly with them. Conceptual skills are about understanding the complexity of the organisation and recognising how what you and the various teams around you do fits with the overall goals of the organisation (e.g. how managing trolley waits in the Emergency Department fits with the overall organisational goal of preventing people waiting longer than necessary anywhere in the hospital).

Managers usually combine all of these skills, but sometimes people at different levels of management use some skills more than others. For instance, a Ward Sister/Charge Nurse is more likely to use more technical and human skills than conceptual ones, whereas the Chief Executive of a hospital would use more conceptual and human skills.

In order to be effective, all managers need to know what and who they are responsible and accountable for.

Medicines management
Definition
Medicines management in the widest sense is 'the clinical, cost-effective and safe use of medicines to ensure patients get the maximum benefit from the medicines they need, while at the same time minimising potential harm' (MHRA, 2004). In NMC (2013 update) Medicines Management Standards. NMC, London.

In nursing, medicines management refers to the prescribing, dispensing, storage, administration and disposal of medicinal products.

(N.B. Students must never engage in any aspect of medicines management without direct supervision.)

Avoiding harm and keeping people safe are vital dimensions of medicines management. In order to achieve them, nurses need to ensure that they comply with the standards of their professional and statutory body. These standards are likely to focus on your involvement in the following:

- Methods of supply and/or administration.
- Checking any direction to administer a medicinal product.
- Storage and transportation.
- Administration of medicines.
- Assessment of the effectiveness of and a patient's response to medicines.
- Assessment of patients who are self-administering medicines or whose carers are doing this.
- Communication with patients about medicines.
- Titration when a range of doses is prescribed to ensure the best response in the patient (e.g. symptom control).
- Preparing medications.
- Use of compliance aids.
- Disposal of medicinal products.
- Delegation and accountability.
- Management of adverse events.
- Reporting of adverse reactions.

As you progress through your nursing course you will gain supervised experience of all aspects of medicines management, so that on registration as a nurse you will be able to adhere to the standards laid down by your professional and statutory body. Some nurses have gained specialist qualifications enabling them to prescribe medicinal products.

As a student, regardless of seniority, you are responsible for reporting patients' adverse reactions to medicinal products immediately, to either a senior nursing colleague or a doctor. Documenting these reactions is essential.

Any deviations from medication plans that you observe should also be reported to your seniors.

Moving and positioning
Definition

Nurses undertake many activities that involve moving and positioning patients (or equipment involved in their care). These include helping a person to move from one place to another, to transfer between their bed and a chair, to change position in bed, or to undertake activities of daily living such as transferring to the toilet, having a bath or shower and dressing.

Inappropriate moving and positioning practice may cause:

* Discomfort and a lack of dignity for the person being moved.
* Accidents that can hurt the person being moved and the person doing the moving.
* Back pain and musculoskeletal disorders for the nurse that can lead to time off work or an inability to continue working in that job.

When you make your initial assessment of a patient, include a risk assessment of their moving and positioning needs. The Health and Safety Executive (HSE, 2013 http://www. hse.gov.uk/healthservices/moving-handling.htm) recommends focusing on:

* the extent of the individual's ability to support their own weight and any other relevant factors, for example pain, disability, spasm, fatigue, tissue viability or tendency to fall;
* the extent to which the individual can participate in/cooperate with transfers;
* whether the individual needs assistance to reposition themselves/sit up when in their bed/chair and how this will be achieved, e.g. provision of an electric profiling bed;
* the specific equipment needed ... and, if applicable, type of bed, bath and chair, as well as specific handling equipment, type of hoist and sling, sling size and attachments;
* the assistance needed for different types of transfer, including the number of staff needed – although hoists can be operated by one person, hoisting tasks often require two staff to ensure safe transfer;
* the arrangements for reducing the risk and for dealing with falls, if the individual is at risk.

Use this risk assessment to plan a person's care and minimise risk to them and to you and your colleagues. Record your assessment for others to use and make sure it is updated when the patient's condition or needs change. In addition to any initial moving and positioning assessment, every time you undertake nursing care make a rapid assessment of any risk involved. Take appropriate action to manage any risk so that no harm will be caused.

To reduce the risks of inappropriate moving and positioning, employers offer regular annual mandatory training. It is important to minimise the risk of undignified care, accidents and harm by adhering to your organisation's manual handling policies and following these principles of good practice.

Always tell colleagues if their moving and positioning practices are deficient.

Practice development
Definition
Practice development is about changing nursing practice to make care better and to improve the environment in which nurses and other members of the multi-disciplinary team work – and of course, within which care is delivered. Practice development is not a new idea: it emerged from the first Nursing Development Units (NDUs), which started developing nursing practice in England in the 1980s. Since then many designated development units have grown up, but you do not need to work in one of these to make improvements to practice – every nurse can do this either as part of their daily individual practice or more collectively as part of the nursing team.

One of the important features of practice development is that it is the people who actually deliver care who are involved in developing practice; it is not a top-down managerial exercise. The essence of sound practice development lies in ownership and involvement, which in turn may lead to feelings of empowerment.

Practice development is a way of thinking *and* working that requires nurses to be innovative and entrepreneurial.

Generally practice development projects need to achieve the following (based on work by McCormack et al., 2006, p. 11):

- Be person centred.
- Work from a clear set of values (e.g. respect, trust, dignity).
- Promote collaboration, participation and shared ownership.
- Use ways to facilitate critical reflection (e.g. action learning).
- Use the best evidence available (usually from research).
- Evaluate the way you did things (process) and the outcomes.
- Use a facilitative and inclusive style to enable change to occur.
- Tell other people what you have done and learnt.

Quality improvement
Definition
In order to ensure that care is the best it can be, services need to be monitored for their quality. This involves informal and formal evaluation – for instance, a nurse and a patient might routinely evaluate care against the goals they have set, or an audit might be carried out on a ward to compare care provided with the local standards expected, or units/ hospitals may be monitored by outside agencies to determine how they meet certain nationally determined standards. Once exercises like this have been done, it is often necessary to improve care.

There are several ways to improve care, but increasingly formal improvement processes such as PDSA (Plan: Do: Study: Act) or LEAN thinking are being used. PDSA is usually used for small-scale change, whereas LEAN thinking is often described as a way of achieving larger-scale change across an organisation(s) or broader health system. These techniques focus on the skills and resources needed to make care better and tailoring these to suit the specific environment within which care needs to be altered.

PDSA was popularised by the Institute for Healthcare Improvement (IHI; http://www.ihi. org/IHI/) in North America and has been used across the world in order to make improvements to healthcare. Essentially, PDSA is about finding the answers to three key questions: What are we trying to accomplish? What change can we make that will result in an improvement? How will we know that a change is an improvement? The cycle is used to 'test a change by developing a plan to test the change (Plan), carrying out the test (Do), observing and learning from the consequences (Study), and determining what modifications should be made to the test (Act)'. The PDSA cycle is most often associated with small-scale change at particular hot spots in an organisation or an individual care pathway. PDSA is useful because it enables you to make a change in care for a group of people or for a ward; if succcessful, these changes can then be scaled up for several similar units or a hospital. PDSA is also useful because it is a bottom-up approach to quality improvement, so once you have decided that something needs to change you can get people involved in order that they own the change. In that way you are more likely to create sustainable change, rather than a short-lived change that no one wants.

Research
Definition
Research is about systematically generating new knowledge to answer specific questions. Nurses need this knowledge to help deliver the best care possible.

There are many different sorts of research designs that help to create new knowledge, such as randomised controlled trials, surveys, case studies, ethnographies and phenomenological studies. Each of these creates different types of data and so gives different answers to research questions. For instance, randomised controlled trials can tell us if an intervention works or not when compared to the usual care, whereas a phenomenological study tells us about people's experiences of care.

Increasingly there is a view that we need to know what works (and does not), why it works and how people feel about it or experience it. To do this, researchers are frequently using more than one method within a study (e.g. mixed-methods designs).

All nurses are expected to be aware of and able to utilise research findings and evaluate their usefulness in everyday practice. Using the most up-to-date and appropriate research and tailoring it to meet the needs of each patient is a fundamental component of skilled, high-quality nursing care.

To use research knowledge effectively, you need to be able to assess the rigour of the research done and its usefulness for practice. This may be daunting, so start by deciding whether there is a good fit between the research question(s) being answered and the question you need an answer to in practice. If there is a good fit, then before deciding to use the research, assess how rigorously it was conducted by asking a few questions. For example:

- Were the research design and methods appropriate for answering the research question?
- Were there enough participants in the study to justify the findings?
- Were threats to validity, reliability and credibility taken into account?
- Have the results been analysed appropriately?
- Do the results answer the research question?
- Are limitations clearly discussed?
- Are the conclusions based on the results and are they justified?

If the research is rigorous and relevant, then the findings can be implemented and evaluated in practice.

Risk assessment and management
Definition

Avoiding harm and keeping people safe are vital dimensions of nursing care. In order to achieve them, nurses need to be able to do the following:

- Identify, assess and report (as necessary) actual and potential threats to a person's safety and health (the risk is the chance that someone might be harmed by one of these threats).
- Understand the cause(s) of these risks and what can be done to lessen them.
- Implement ways to avoid, reduce or control them (management).
- Evaluate the success of their actions.

Risks could include a patient's likelihood of falling at home, of taking the wrong medication at the wrong time if self-medicating, of acquiring an infection while in hospital or of developing a venous thromboembolism after a period of inactivity.

Organisational policies and procedures guide the assessment and management of risks to patients, their families/carers, colleagues and yourself. Sometimes checklists (e.g. pre-operatively) or risk measurement scales (e.g. for assessing the risk of developing pressure ulcers) are used to ensure that risks are assessed and minimised.

Risk management is a term also used by organisations to describe the structures and processes they have put in place and use to identify and manage risk.

Patient safety incidents are unintended or unforeseen events that could have harmed or did harm a patient. These should always be taken seriously and investigated to work out what went wrong and what could be done to stop the same thing happening again. Learning from this analysis is important. This process should usually be blame free.

Knowing the part you play in maintaining patient safety is critical – a good example of this is the relationship between thorough hand washing and infection control. Being mindful of the safety of colleagues and yourself is also important. If you think that a patient or a colleague is at risk, tell an appropriate person.

Teamwork
Definition
Teamwork can simply be defined as working with other people to achieve a common goal. In healthcare teamwork can encompass many things, including working with other professionals in multi-disciplinary or inter-professional teams; working across agencies in inter-agency collaborations (e.g. healthcare, social care and housing); working with patients, their family and their friends; or working with other nurses in a uni-professional team. Whatever the sort of team, streamlined, coordinated care is the goal.

Nurses fit into this complex system of teams in a variety of different ways, ranging from facilitating the complicated negotiation of services and treatments to maintaining routine functioning for a patient. Nurses are often seen as the key people who help others navigate their way around care and services.

Effective teamwork involves the following aspects:

- Ensuring that the right people are part of the team – this means that the patient and their family are always involved.
- Making sure that everyone understands the goals the team is trying to achieve.
- Matching the skills and knowledge of team members to these goals.
- Ensuring that everyone knows what is expected of them.
- Creating an environment within which people trust each other and are able to clarify their responsibilities and take decisions collaboratively and independently within explicit boundaries.
- Ensuring that everyone can voice concerns and be supported in their work.
- Making sure that communication is clear within and outwith the team.
- Giving the team members opportunities to meet and review their work so they can make improvements as care is delivered.
- Enabling the team to celebrate success and examine areas for improvement in a non-judgemental way.

Wound management
Definition
Wound management is a very important aspect of nursing in the hospital and the community. Wounds may be deliberately formed (surgical incisions) or be the result of injury (accident) or a complication of illness (e.g. diabetes) or altered circulation (leg ulcers), which may sometimes be coupled with pressure (e.g. pressure ulcers). Wounds can be acute (short lived) or chronic (long term).

Wound healing can be achieved in a number of different ways, for instance:

- The edges of a wound can be joined together by sutures, staples or other forms of closure (healing by primary intention).
- If wound edges cannot be brought together, the wound is left to heal through contraction and epithelialisation (healing by secondary intention).
- The edges of some wounds cannot be joined immediately and will be left for a short time before joining (healing by tertiary intention).

There are four broad phases to wound healing: haemostasis, inflammation, proliferation/epithelialisation and maturation, when the wound becomes strengthened and scar tissue is formed, thins and fades.

Wound healing can be delayed by poor nutrition, alterations in temperature, ongoing excess exudate, poor dressing (or inappropriate) technique or use of the wrong dressings. During all procedures associated with wounds (e.g. dressing, drain emptying or removal, suture removal) nurses must ensure that they protect patients, through asepsis, against acquired infections.

The principles of wound management include:

- Making sure that the patient knows when you are going to change dressings and that suitable analgesia has been given beforehand.
- Ensuring privacy.
- Picking the right dressings for the wound (e.g. alginates, occlusive, hydrocolloid, hydrogel, foams).
- Choosing the right cleansing agents.
- Ensuring that you have all the equipment needed before starting to expose the wound.
- Remembering hand washing/cleansing with antibacterial substances and asepsis throughout the procedure.
- Evaluating the wound every time a dressing is changed (Dougherty & Lister, 2011) and recording:
  - Size
  - Wound bed (necrotic – black, slough – yellow, granulating – red, epithelialising – pink)
  - Skin around the wound (e.g. intact, healthy, inflamed – allergy to dressing/tape)
  - Exudate (amount)
  - Odour
  - Bleeding
  - Pain
  - Infection (take swab)
- Recording observations and communicating any concerns to a senior member of the team.

Part 2   Conditions

Acute coronary syndromes

Definition

Unstable angina (UA) and heart attacks (myocardial infarctions, MI) are referred to as acute coronary syndromes (ACS) and are medical emergencies.

Their common pathology is sudden total/near total blockage of a coronary vessel, usually due to atherosclerotic plaque rupture leading to an intracoronary thrombus. The blockage may be episodic or transient (UA) or complete, resulting in reduced blood flow or complete blockage and the death of some of the myocardium (MI). Presentation and treatment depend on where the blockage is and whether it is complete or partial. MI are managed according to their type – ST elevation myocardial infarctions (STEMI) or non-ST segment elevation myocardial infarctions (NSTEMI). *STEMI* shows sustained elevation of the ST segments of the ECG, indicating a large area of myocardium death. Troponins are elevated (troponins are proteins found in heart muscle and damage causes specific troponins to leak out into the bloodstream). *NSTEMI* causes less myocardial damage so may not cause ST elevation, but elevated troponins are present. There may be other ECG changes, such as ST depression or T-wave inversion.

UA manifests as ACS symptoms, but there is no ST elevation/raised troponins. UA results in ischaemia, but no destruction of myocardium.

Diagnosis and investigations

Diagnosis is made by examination, history taking, 12-lead ECGs to identify STEMI/NSTEMI/UA, and blood tests to assess myocardial damage (e.g. troponins T and I).

Common signs and symptoms

Pain usually at rest; unrelieved by nitrovasodilators; continuous and lasts longer than 15 minutes; described as crushing, tight or constricting; may radiate to arms and neck (may be described in the stomach area); sometimes no pain at all. Fear. Pallor and/or sweaty or clammy skin; cyanosis. Sometimes shortness of breath; nausea and vomiting; altered level of consciousness. Change in heart rate (usually tachycardia), rhythm and blood pressure (BP).

Treatment

In the acute phase management focuses on symptom control (pain relief usually with diamorphine, antiemetics to reduce nausea and oxygen if hypoxic), improving blood flow to the heart and reducing demand for oxygen by rest and drug therapy.

STEMI treatment focuses on reperfusion/revascularisation, either pharmacological (thrombolysis) or by percutaneous coronary intervention (PCI) – balloon catheter passed into coronary artery, balloon inflated to open narrowed vessel, stent inserted.

NSTEMI and UA are treated pharmacologically, for instance by antiplatelet therapy (e.g. aspirin), antithrombin therapy (e.g. low molecular weight heparin). Beta-blockers and nitrates are used if needed.

Both conditions can progress to STEMI.

Following the acute phase attention focuses on education, rehabilitation, secondary prevention (e.g. long-term aspirin, statin use) and cardiac interventions (e.g. revascularisation).

Nursing care

Providing highly skilled nursing care for people with MI is critical to their recovery. Many different nurses may be involved in a person's care pathway, depending on where the patient presents with symptoms. Immediate care will focus on assessing pain levels, nausea and anxiety, giving medications/oxygen as prescribed, and monitoring and reporting the person's condition (e.g. alterations in heart rate, fall in blood pressure, decreasing blood oxygen saturation, restlessness, breathlessness, falling pulse pressure). Reassuring communication with an explanation of interventions, equipment and plans will reduce anxiety. As recovery progresses, discuss with the patient suitable activity levels and monitor the effects of resumption of activity. Nurses may also be responsible for ongoing monitoring and health education and promotion once the patient is discharged from hospital.

Acute renal failure
Definition
Acute renal failure is a syndrome characterised by rapid decline (days to weeks) in glomerular filtration rate (GFR). This results in an accumulation of nitrogenous waste and problems regulating extracellular volume and electrolytes. Urine output may be reduced (oliguria) or non-existent (anuria).

The kidneys comprise three parts: the renal cortex, the renal medulla and the renal pelvis. Kidneys primarily separate waste and excess water from blood and convert this filtrate into urine (filtration, selective reabsorption and secretion). Filtration occurs in the glomeruli (glomerular filtration). The glomeruli filter around 7 L of fluid/hour producing 50–100 ml of urine. Substances needed to maintain acid base and fluid balance are reabsorbed from the filtrate by osmosis, diffusion and active transportation. Ions, creatinine, urea and some hormones are secreted. Urine is stored in the bladder until it leaves the body via the urethra. Antidiuretic hormone (ADH) regulates the amount of urine passed.

The kidneys also have an endocrine function synthesising hormones. Renin and angiotensin regulate sodium and fluid retention and the expansion and contraction of blood vessels, and have a role in BP control. Renin controls the glomerular blood flow and filtration rate.

Acute renal failure results from a variety of causes (pre-renal, renal and post-renal). Pre-renal causes largely relate to hypo-perfusion of the kidneys. This mainly stems from other system failures, for instance cardiovascular. Renal causes result from diseases affecting the kidney. Post-renal causes are associated with urinary tract obstructions. Disruption to the functioning of the kidneys will affect many bodily functions and systems.

Diagnosis and investigations
Patients with acute renal failure may present with a range of signs and symptoms, including oliguria/anuria, nausea/vomiting, malaise, hypertension, peripheral oedema, breathlessness (pulmonary oedema/metabolic acidosis), pericarditis, encephalopathy and hyperkalaemia. Investigations will include urinalysis, kidney function and blood tests.

Treatment
Treatment focuses on ensuring adequate oxygenation and circulation, and management of the presenting symptoms and the underlying causes. Dialysis (renal replacement therapy) may be required. Acute renal failure may be reversible.

Nursing care
Restoring and maintaining homeostasis are central aspects of care. This will involve careful monitoring of fluid balance and skilled observation of the patient's condition for deterioration (or improvement). Focus on:

- Urinalysis (look for protein, blood, cells and casts).
- Fluid balance: intake and output measurement (over- or under-hydration).
- Oxygen saturation and respiratory rate.
- Oxygen administration, recording and monitoring.
- Alterations in heart rate, rhythm and blood pressure.
- ECG: cardiac arrhythmias due to hyperkalaemia.
- Alteration in level of consciousness.
- Nutritional status/hydration (enteral/parenteral feeding may be needed).
- Signs of oedema in peripheral tissues due to fluid and electrolyte disruption.
- Compromised skin (oedema, waterlogged tissues at risk of infection).
- Signs of infection (redness around IVI sites, pyrexia).

Acute renal failure can be very frightening, so accurate, explanatory and empathic communication is essential.

Anaemias
Definition
WHO (http://www.who.int/nutrition/publications/micronutrients/global_prevalence_anaemia_2011/en/) defined anaemia as less than 12 g/dL Hb for non-pregnant women, less than 11 g/dL Hb for pregnant women and less than 13 g/dL Hb for men. Haemoglobin (Hb) levels normally vary between individuals. Women tend to have lower levels than men. There are various types of anaemia (e.g. iron-deficiency anaemia, thalassaemia, aplastic anaemia, pernicious anaemia and haemolytic anaemia).

Anaemia occurs because there are insufficient/poorly functioning red blood cells (RBC) or there is a reduction in haemoglobin in each RBC. Reduced haemoglobin means that RBC carry less oxygen. Anaemias are usually classified according to RBC size – microcytic/hypochromic (small red blood cells with less haemoglobin than normal); normochromic/normocytic (normal haemoglobin, normal-sized red blood cells); or macrocytic (red blood cells are larger than normal).

Anaemias are caused by different illnesses/deficiencies. Iron deficiency is the most common cause of anaemia in the world. *Iron-deficiency anaemia* may occur because of blood loss (e.g. through menstruation, gastro-intestinal [GI] bleeding), an iron-deficient diet, pregnancy, poor absorption of iron (e.g. coeliac disease) or hookworm infection. In *pernicious anaemia* vitamin B12 cannot be absorbed. Antibodies are formed against intrinsic factor (IF) or against the cells in the stomach that make IF, which stops IF from attaching to vitamin B12 and prevents its absorption. *Thalassaemia* is a genetic condition that affects the alpha or beta chains of haemoglobin. Consequently there is insufficient normal haemoglobin and the red blood cells break down easily. Thalassaemia is part of the group of *haemolytic anaemias* (also including sickle cell disease) where red blood cell life is shortened. *Aplastic anaemia* is a disorder of the bone marrow resulting in a deficiency of all blood cells.

Diagnosis and investigations
Diagnosis is made by examination, history and blood tests, for instance full blood count, haemoglobin concentration, haematocrit (or packed cell volume, PCV), blood film. Bone marrow examination and other specific tests will also be done for some people.

Common signs and symptoms
Symptoms and signs depend on underlying pathologies, but may include tiredness, peripheral oedema such as swollen feet, breathlessness, feeling faint, angina if there are underlying heart problems, pallor in conjunctiva, or spoon-shaped nails in long-standing anaemia.

Treatment
Treatment is of the underlying disease. It may include hospitalisation or be carried out in primary care. Options include iron supplements (and dietary advice), blood transfusion, recombinant erythropoietin and vitamin supplements/replacements.

Nursing care
The nursing care of people with anaemia will depend on the severity of their disease and its underlying pathology. For some people no treatment will be required except for advice about dietary changes (e.g. eating food rich in iron and also ensuring an adequate intake of vitamin C – which may help the body to absorb iron – and protein); for others iron or vitamin B12 supplements may be prescribed; in severe cases some people will need blood transfusions. Hypoxia related to anaemia may cause tiredness, breathlessness and associated anxiety. Advice should be given about how to alleviate each of these, for example making sure that rest is planned into daily routines may help with controlling tiredness and breathlessness; sitting upright also may assist with reducing feelings of breathlessness. Some people may also report a sore mouth, which will affect their appetite, and an oral assessment should be carried out if this is the case. Smoking can have an impact on anaemia, so smoking cessation should be discussed and supported.

Aneurysms
Definition
An aneurysm is a permanent local dilatation of an artery. The affected artery may be 1.5 times its normal diameter. Aneurysms can occur in the abdominal aorta and the iliac, femoral and popliteal arteries. Cerebral and thoracic aneurysms are less common. Abdominal aortic aneurysms (AAA) are the most common. A high degree of mortality (around 85%) is associated with a ruptured AAA.

Diagnosis, screening and investigations
History/presentation – pulsating mass; local organ pain due to pressure from aneurysm.
    Ultrasound/CT scan. Risk factors include smoking, atherosclerosis, hypertension and hyperlipidaemia, so assessment for these should be included.
    AAA screening can be done by ultrasound and is available to men over 65, as AAA is more common in men than in women. If an AAA is present then careful monitoring is needed to enable intervention to be planned electively.

Treatment
Treatment is usually by endovascular aneurysm repair (EVAR), for example stent insertion, or surgical repair with graft; no medical treatment is possible. If repair is successful then there is a good prognosis.

Nursing care
Aneurysms are frightening and patients and their families will need reassurance and psychological support. For those whose aneurysms have been detected at screening or before rupture, careful monitoring and assessment will occur as an outpatient prior to elective surgery or EVAR. For those with sudden rupture of an aneurysm, emergency surgery is necessary. In the case of a ruptured AAA nursing care will focus on stabilising BP, largely by infusion of blood expanders, medication administration and preparation for emergency surgery.
    For people admitted for elective repair of aneurysms, nursing care will revolve around the following:

- Reassuring the patient and family about procedures and what to expect post-operatively.
- Monitoring vital signs regularly post-operatively, especially for hypovolaemic shock, hypertension, infection, arrhythmias and breathing problems.
- Assessing and monitoring limb perfusion regularly (hourly).
- Monitoring the wound site for haemorrhage and any drain. Abdominal girth measurements may be needed to check for signs of expansion due to haemorrhage.
- Encouraging passive leg movement to increase perfusion and reduce risk of DVT. Also deep breathing.
- Ensuring pressure-relieving equipment is used.
- Focusing on pain assessment and management, making sure that the patient and family report pain.
- Focusing on assessment of anxiety; discuss worries and if necessary possible night sedation with the doctor.
- Increasing mobility and independence depending on rate of recovery.
- Providing ongoing reassurance and health promotion and education.

Angina
Definition

Angina is a dull, heavy or tight pain/discomfort in the chest, sometimes radiating to the arm, neck, jaw or back. It occurs when the blood supply to the muscles of the heart is restricted. There are two types of angina: stable and unstable. In stable angina the pain is usually triggered by exercise or stress and lasts only a few minutes, normally resolving once the trigger has been removed (or medication taken). In unstable angina the attack does not necessarily have an obvious trigger and does not resolve with rest – this sort of angina attack requires emergency medical attention (see Acute coronary syndromes).

Diagnosis and investigations

History and examination.

Treatment

Treatment for stable angina is usually taken when the pain occurs and consists of glyceryl trinitrate (either a spray or a tablet dissolved under the tongue). Some people will also be treated with, for example, beta-blockers or calcium channel blockers.

Nursing care

Knowing that someone has angina is important when they are liable to become stressed, as is the case if they are in hospital. Being able to reassure them and give them appropriate medication (glyceryl trinitrate) is important. It is also important to be able to recognise if stable angina becomes unstable and to call for immediate medical help.

Most people with angina are cared for in the community. Practice nurses and community nurses will be involved in monitoring the patient's condition as well as giving appropriate advice about such issues as exercise, stress reduction, diet and weight.

Appendicitis

Definition
Appendicitis is an inflammation of the vermiform appendix usually associated with blockage of the lumen. It is a common surgical emergency. Removal of the appendix (appendicectomy) can be performed either as open surgery or using a laparoscope. Complications may include perforation, abscess formation and peritonitis. Intravenous antibiotic therapy will be needed if the appendix has perforated.

Diagnosis and investigations
History and examination.

Common signs and symptoms
Abdominal pain that eventually settles at the lower right-hand side. Pressing, coughing or walking can make the pain worse. Nausea and vomiting (sometimes diarrhoea) and loss of appetite. Pyrexia.

Treatment
Appendicectomy.

Nursing care
Appendicitis is a medical emergency. Operating before the appendix ruptures and causes peritonitis is the critical concern. People admitted to hospital with appendicitis will be generally fit but acutely ill. Accurate assessment and monitoring are essential to recognise signs of perforation and peritonitis (e.g. increased pain, abdominal rigidity, pyrexia, vomiting, extreme weakness and shock); these should be reported to senior colleagues or a doctor. If such symptoms persist post-operatively, an abdominal abscess may have developed.

Arrhythmias
Definition
Normal heart rhythm is called sinus rhythm. The usual number of heart beats in sinus rhythm is between 60 and 100 at rest. If this regular rhythm is faster than 100 it is sinus tachycardia; if slower than 60 it is sinus bradycardia.

Arrhythmias are abnormal heart beats caused by irregularities in the electrical conduction system of the heart. They lead to an irregular pulse and can be seen on ECG tracings as disturbance in the usual PQRST wave. Arrhythmias can cause alterations in heart rate, myocardial oxygen requirement and blood flow.

Arrhythmias can either be fast (tachyarrhythmia) or slow (bradyarrhythmia).

Tachyarrhythmias include atrial flutter, atrial fibrillation, ventricular tachycardia and ventricular fibrillation.

Bradyarrhythmias include sinus bradycardia or sinus arrest, bundle branch block and atrioventricular block.

Minor arrhythmias are common and usually unproblematic. Sometimes they are due to extra (ectopic) heart beats followed by a slight pause before the next beat. The person might feel this as a palpitation.

However, some arrhythmias can compromise cardiac function and cause sudden death, such as ventricular tachycardia or ventricular fibrillation.

Diagnosis and investigations
Physical examination and history taking. 12-lead ECGs.

Common signs and symptoms
Although serious arrhythmias can be asymptomatic, patients often experience arrhythmias as dizziness, feeling faint or fainting (syncope), shortness of breath, chest pain, headache or being unable to sustain usual levels of activity.

Treatment
The consequences of arrhythmias vary and often one arrhythmia can progress to a more serious type – for instance, atrial flutter to atrial fibrillation; ventricular tachycardia to ventricular fibrillation. Careful assessment and monitoring of ECGs are therefore vital together with close observation for symptoms. Treatment will depend on the arrhythmia.

Nursing care
A patient may develop an arrhythmia while in hospital or be admitted with one. Every nurse should be able to recognise a normal ECG pattern and deviation from it. Nursing care centres on monitoring the patient's condition, their response to treatment of the arrhythmia and any underlying conditions, such as coronary heart disease (CHD).

Asthma
Definition
Clinically asthma is said to be present if a combination of cough, wheeze or breathlessness occurs with variable airflow obstruction. Airway obstruction is reversible. Asthma is a chronic condition with acute exacerbations.

Asthma can be divided into three groups: extrinsic, intrinsic and occupational.

Extrinsic asthma is common in childhood and largely triggered by allergens (e.g. dust mites, animal hair/fur, pollen). Allergens are inhaled and absorbed by the bronchial mucosa, triggering an inflammatory reaction that results in bronchial muscle spasm, oedema and secretion of thick mucus. Asthma attacks may lessen with age and good management.

Intrinsic asthma develops later in life and is less likely to be caused by allergens. Intrinsic asthma may respond less well to treatment than extrinsic asthma.

Occupational asthma is caused by workplace allergens.

Exercise, cold air, high atmospheric ozone (e.g. in thunderstorms), viral infections and emotional stress can also trigger asthma attacks.

Diagnosis and investigations
History taking and examination. Lung function tests to show airflow obstruction. Serial peak flow measurements may show a pattern of morning dips and night-time peaks of peak expiratory flow rate (PEFR). Peak flow measurements are important markers of severity once asthma has been diagnosed.

Common signs and symptoms
A person with asthma may have one or more of cough, wheezing, chest tightness and breathlessness.

Being unable to complete a sentence in one breath is a serious warning sign – call for immediate medical help.

Treatment
Can include bronchodilators, inhaled/oral steroids and leukotriene receptor antagonists/ theophyllines.

Identifying triggers and reducing contact with them are also important.

Nursing care
Most nursing care for patients with asthma will be undertaken in primary care by practice nurses, who regularly monitor a patient's medication regimes, lung function and attack frequency. If a patient's asthma is not well controlled, the practice nurse will consult the GP and advise a review. Practice nurses will provide advice about medications and inhaler techniques, avoidance of triggers, recognising the severity of asthma attacks and knowing when to seek medical help.

If a patient is admitted to hospital with a severe asthma attack, highly skilled, observant nursing is needed: a patient's condition can quickly deteriorate and severe asthma attacks can be life threatening. In this instance the aim of treatment is to minimise hypoxia and reduce bronchoconstriction and airway inflammation. Treatment with oxygen therapy, corticosteroids and nebulised bronchodilators will be started immediately.

Breast lumps
Definition
A breast lump is a palpable mass in the breast. Breast lumps are a common but much feared occurrence in women. They are uncommon in men.

Breast lumps are due to a number of causes in women: fibroadenoma, localised benign fibrocystic disease, cysts and cancer.

In men enlargement of the breast may cause concern, but may not in itself have serious health consequences. Breast enlargement is largely due to hyperplasia of glandular tissue caused by, for instance, obesity, hyperprolactinaemia (high level of prolactin), systemic disease such as liver cirrhosis, chronic renal failure or an underlying hormone-secreting tumour. However, men can get breast cancer, although rarely, so any enlargement of breasts and the presence of lumps, alterations to nipples or skin texture should be investigated.

Diagnosis, screening and investigations
Clinical examination and history; imaging (ultrasound, mammography, magnetic resonance imaging [MRI] scan); fine needle aspiration cytology/biopsy.

Treatment
The treatment of benign breast lumps depends on their cause, for example cysts may need draining.

The treatment of breast cancer will depend on the results of disease staging, type of cancer and discussions with the patient and their family/carers about their preferred treatment. The options will include mastectomy and restoration of the breast, lumpectomy and breast-conserving surgery, followed by chemotherapy/radiotherapy. Sometimes ovaries are also removed (oophorectomy).

Nursing care
Anyone having a breast lump investigated will require sensitive, informative care that helps to alleviate anxiety. If breast cancer is diagnosed, the person and their family will benefit from reassuring, honest communication to enable them to deal with not only the diagnosis of cancer, but also an inevitable change in body image. They may wish to discuss all treatment possibilities with practice nurses, specialist breast care nurses, GPs and consultant oncologists/breast surgeons before coming to a final decision about treatment. Some cancer will be hereditary and so there will be an extra concern of passing the faulty gene onto children. Genetic counselling may be recommended.

If surgery is needed, recovery will depend on the type of surgery performed and the subsequent outcome with regard to the need for chemotherapy and/or radiotherapy. Nursing care will then need to focus on these treatments and their associated side effects, as well as supporting the patient (and their family/carers) emotionally and psychologically.

Breathlessness
Definition

Breathlessness (dyspnoea) occurs when someone has difficulty breathing. It is a very frightening and debilitating symptom, which can be acute or chronic.

Both acute and chronic breathlessness are largely attributed to cardiac and/or pulmonary causes, but acute breathlessness may also be caused by pain, diabetic ketoacidosis, drug overdoses (e.g. aspirin), trauma or altitude sickness. Chronic breathlessness may be caused by severe anaemia, anxiety, thromboembolic disease, obesity or thyroid disease.

Hyperventilation is sometimes known as behavioural breathlessness. The management of hyperventilation is different to the management of breathlessness described here and involves careful explanation of the situation, a calm manner to relieve anxiety, rebreathing using a paper bag or cupped hands if hyperventilation has been confirmed. Relaxation techniques can be helpful.

Diagnosis and investigations

Breathlessness can be assessed using the MRC Dyspnoea Scale:

Grade	Degree of breathlessness related to activities
1	Not troubled by breathlessness except on strenuous exercise
2	Short of breath when hurrying or walking up a slight hill
3	Walks slower than contemporaries on level ground because of breathlessness; or has to stop for breath when walking at own pace
4	Stops for breath after walking about 100 m or after a few minutes on level ground
5	Too breathless to leave the house, or breathless when dressing or undressing

Nursing care

- Find out more about the current episode of breathlessness. Ask about any triggers and whether anything in particular relieves breathlessness – important in chronic breathlessness.
- Assess the general level of distress that the breathlessness is causing: colour of skin, cyanosis, pallor, clamminess, respiratory rate and quality, pulse.
- Call for medical advice if there has been a new acute episode or worsening of the patient's condition.
- Reassure the patient and explain simply and clearly what is happening and what you would like them to do.
- If the patient is prescribed oxygen or drugs to reduce breathlessness, make sure these are given immediately you become aware of the symptoms. Evaluate the success (or not) of these interventions and report this to a senior colleague or doctor.
- If appropriate, loosen any restricting clothing that the patient is wearing.
- Ask the patient to sit in a more upright position (this may require your assistance and repositioning the pillows and backrest). Sometimes leaning slightly forward is useful too, using a table/bed table as a support.
- Consider using controlled breathing techniques: ask the patient to focus on their breathing to make it slower and deeper. Ask them to relax their shoulders and upper chest to reduce fast, ineffective and shallow breathing. Sometimes patients will be able to do this more effectively if you also do the same thing: sitting at their level, talking them through each action and doing it so that they can mirror your behaviour.
- If breathlessness continues once an acute episode has subsided, consider how to adapt activities of daily living to suit the patient. Discuss with colleagues and patient's family/carers.
- Discuss lifestyle modifications at an appropriate time (e.g. exercise, smoking cessation, weight and diet).

Cancer
Definition
Cancer occurs when normal cells grow uncontrollably (e.g. as a tumour), damaging or destroying the tissue of origin and infiltrating and destroying neighbouring organs and tissues. Unlike other cells, cancer uses the blood and lymph systems to spread and grow in other parts of the body (metastasise). Cells may become cancerous (malignant) as a result of exposure to various factors, including chemicals, radiation, viruses or other organisms, and through heredity. Cancer can affect any of the body's systems and there are over 200 different types of cancer. The most common cancers in the UK are found in the lungs, bowel, breasts and prostate gland. The consequences of cancer are wide-ranging and vary from complete cure to long-term management to rapid death. Around 25% of all deaths are caused by cancer. However, many people live with cancer for years and do not die from it.

Prevention and early detection
Some cancers can be prevented, including lung cancer (smoking cessation), malignant melanoma (protection from sunshine), cervical cancer (immunisation; condom use) and some mouth cancers (dietary modification). Screening is an important way to identify cancers early, for instance for cervical cancer through smear tests, colorectal cancer through testing for faecal occult blood or breast cancer through mammography.

Diagnosis, screening and investigations
As cancer manifests itself in different ways depending on its location, stage of development and the person's overall health, signs and symptoms associated with cancer will vary and so in turn will nursing care. The early diagnosis of cancer is an important aspect of successful treatment and so symptom recognition is central to many cancer awareness campaigns. Patients who are experiencing unusual signs and symptoms, such as unusual bleeding, altered routines (for instance bowel habits), nausea, loss of appetite, lumps, pain, fatigue, breathlessness or unintended weight loss, should be referred to their GP, practice nurse or specialist cancer nurse.

Treatment
The treatment and management of cancer have improved significantly, with the result that more people than before are now surviving cancer. There are many different ways to treat and manage cancer (e.g. surgery, chemotherapy, radiotherapy, immunotherapy, monoclonal antibodies or a combination of treatments). Cancer treatments may cause a number of side effects, some that are unpleasant (e.g. nausea, vomiting, hair loss, fatigue, lymphodema) and others that are dangerous (e.g. neutropenia).

Nursing care
Integrated, person-centred, multi-disciplinary, multi-agency care is essential regardless of the type, stage or location of the cancer. The nursing care of people with cancer will vary from person to person and also for each person and their family/carers as their cancer progresses, remits or is cured. Nurses will care for people with cancer and their families/carers in many situations and in any setting where healthcare is delivered. The increased survival rate means that nurses' attention needs to focus on treatment management *and* on supporting people to live with (or with having had) cancer so that patients are able to make the necessary adjustments to their life and retain confidence and control of their health and quality of life.

Having (or having had) cancer can leave a person with feelings of loss, altered body image, anxiety, uncertainty and fear of recurrence. Help with psychological as well as physical adjustment to cancer is an important facet of nursing care.

When cancer is terminal, attention needs to switch seamlessly from treatment to palliation and when appropriate to end-of-life care.

Cardiovascular disorders
Definition
The cardiovascular system comprises the heart and blood vessels. Disorders of this system are called cardiovascular disease (CVD) and can result in acute or chronic conditions. The main disorders of the heart are associated with blockage of the coronary arteries, heart muscle damage, altered electrical activity, valve disease or infection. The main disorders of the blood vessels result from atheroma, dysfunctional venous valves and aneurysm. Over 75% of CVD deaths are in low- and middle-income countries (http://www.who.int/mediacentre/factsheets/fs317/en/).

Common cardiovascular disorders include hypertension, coronary heart disease, acute coronary syndromes (unstable angina and heart attack), chronic coronary syndromes, heart failure, valve diseases, arrhythmias, aneurysm and peripheral vascular disease.

Diagnosis, screening and investigations
These will vary depending on the disorder, but are likely to include history taking and examination, ECG and blood tests.

Treatment
This will depend on the disorder.

Nursing care
The nursing of someone with a cardiovascular disorder will depend on the disorder and their state of health. However, accurate assessment and monitoring are vital elements of nursing care. Assessment of the cardiovascular system involves monitoring the following (based on Dougherty & Lister, 2011):

- Pulse – count rate (normal range 55–90/min); feel rhythm (normally regular sequence) and amplitude (strength) for 60 seconds.
- Apical beat – listen with stethoscope; compare rate with radial pulse in patients with atrial fibrillation.
- Blood pressure (BP) – normal range 110–140 mmHg systolic/70–90 mmHg diastolic. Taken electronically or manually.
- Electrical activity of the heart – 12-lead ECG usually in hospital; ambulatory in community.
- Pulse oximetry – electronic probe positioned on end of finger gives pulse rate and oxygen saturation (normal 95–100%).
- Skin colour and condition (e.g. flushed, pallor, cyanosis; dry, cold, warm, sweaty, clammy).
- Central venous pressure (if appropriate).
- Respiratory function – rate, depth and effort (the MRC breathlessness scale may be useful).
- Urine output.
- Mental state – anxiety, level of confusion (incorrect responses to questions) or new disorientation related to self, time and/or place.
- Level of consciousness (the Glasgow Coma Scale may be used).
- Distress and fatigue.
- Find out more about the patient's lifestyle, for instance diet, exercise, alcohol consumption and smoking.
- Find out more about their family history in relation to cardiovascular disease.

Cataracts

Definition

Cataracts form when the lens of the eye becomes opaque as a result of ageing/trauma/ disease (e.g. diabetes). Cataracts are common, particularly in older age, so nurses will frequently care for a person with cataracts. Being aware of their effects is therefore important.

Seeing through a cataract is often described as looking through a frosted window (e.g. a gradual dimming, reduced distance vision and alterations to colour and depth perception). These alterations will have an impact on a person's usual activities, making some routines difficult (e.g. reading small print, seeing the edge of stairs, feeling confident walking in unfamiliar places).

Diagnosis

Eye examination by an ophthalmologist or optometrist.

Treatment

Replacing the opaque lens with an artificial lens (intraocular lens implantation) under a local anaesthetic is the preferred treatment.

Nursing care

Lens replacement usually requires a short stay in hospital as a day patient, preceded by pre-operative assessment of the eye and general health. After the operation, ongoing care at home is focused on the instillation of eye drops (usually by the patient, although some people will require extra help to do this effectively).

Cholecystitis
Definition
Inflammation of the gall bladder is called cholecystitis. It can be caused by either a blockage of the cystic duct in the gallbladder by a gallstone/biliary sludge (calculous cholecystitis), or by infection/injury that damages the gallbladder (acalculous cholecystitis).

Diagnosis and investigations
History: signs and symptoms include persistent pain (sudden and severe or grumbling) in the right upper quadrant of the abdomen (often brought on by fatty food); nausea, vomiting; fever if infection; loss of appetite; obstructive jaundice (cholestatic jaundice) with pale stools and orange urine (biliary obstruction) may occur.

Abdominal examination, blood tests and ultrasound abdominal scan.

Treatment
Hospitalisation is highly likely.

Fasting to protect the gallbladder from further strain, intravenous fluids to prevent dehydration and pain relief. If an infection is suspected antibiotics will be given.

Recurrent cholecystitis may require the removal of the gallbladder (cholecystectomy), through either keyhole or open surgery.

Nursing care
Pain, nausea and vomiting are likely to be the patient's dominant problems. Nurses also need to monitor the patient for signs of hypovolaemic shock (due to excessive vomiting, pain) and infection (pyrexia and tachycardia). Careful assessment of fluid balance and response to medication is required. Be attentive for signs of obstructive jaundice (pale stools and orange urine). Surgical removal of the gall bladder (cholecystectomy) may be needed, in which case attention to pre- and post-operative care is required.

Chronic obstructive pulmonary disease
Definition
Chronic obstructive pulmonary disease (COPD) is a chronic, slowly progressing disorder characterised by fixed or partially reversible airway obstruction. There is no cure for COPD, but skilled management of symptoms can slow its progress. Lifestyle changes and medication can improve health and wellbeing.

COPD is most common in industrialised countries and inner cities, in people who have worked in jobs where they have been exposed to noxious substances and in older people. Cigarette smoking can result in COPD; smoking cessation is strongly advised and can considerably improve COPD. Many people with COPD have never smoked, however. COPD affects 1 in 8 middle-aged and older adults in the UK and accounts for around 5% of UK deaths each year.

Diagnosis and investigations
Physical examination, history taking (symptoms of COPD include cough and shortness of breath, particularly on exertion; sputum may also be present) and spirometry. The severity of COPD is defined by the degree of airflow obstruction (Forced Expiratory Volume in 1 s, FEV1). Flow in *and* out of the lungs is impeded.

Treatment
Treatment may include long-term oxygen therapy (LTOT) for people with chronic hypoxaemia; LTOT is low-dose oxygen given for around 16 hours each day, usually overnight. (N.B. A high percentage of oxygen may reduce respiratory drive.) There may also be pulmonary rehabilitation (exercise training, breathing control, disease education, nutritional advice and social/psychological support) to improve symptoms and the person's quality of life.

Treatment of acute exacerbations may involve bronchodilators, antibiotics and oral corticosteroids. Prescribed oxygen therapy will be in conjunction with arterial blood gas (ABG) monitoring and pulse oximetry.

Nursing care
Management of COPD is largely about lifestyle change and medication adherence. Acute episodes may require hospitalisation. If a patient is admitted to hospital with severe exacerbation of COPD, highly skilled, observant nursing is required. Exacerbation of COPD can lead to respiratory failure. Nurses need to be alert to signs and symptoms of respiratory failure (e.g. restlessness, confusion, increased rate of breathing with greater effort and use of respiratory and abdominal muscles, changed pattern of breathing, flaring of the nostrils, pale or cyanosed clammy skin). Physiotherapy will be important too.

In terms of lifestyle modification, stopping smoking is of the greatest importance, so smoking cessation advice and support should be given. Taking more general exercise (up to 20 minutes a day) will improve patients' COPD symptoms and help them to feel better. This may be hard at first because exercise causes breathlessness; if this happens, stopping the exercise, recovering and then continuing are advised. Eating well is important – dietary advice should be given and weight reviewed (both overweight and underweight). Referral to a dietician might be needed. Recognising exacerbations so they can be treated quickly is very important. Things to look out for include worsened breathlessness and cough (with or without sputum). Inhalers may seem less effective. Fever and generally feeling off colour or tired may also be some of the first symptoms experienced.

Sometimes people with COPD feel anxious or depressed, so careful assessment of their mood is important – remember to allow time to talk about their problems, give reassurance and refer on if extra psychological support is needed.

Chronic renal failure
Definition
Chronic renal failure (CRF) is defined as a consistently, abnormally low glomerular filtration rate (GFR) for more than three months. Chronic renal failure results from a variety of causes (e.g. diabetes mellitus, polycystic kidney disease, obstructive uropathy). There is no cure for CRF. Chronic renal failure means that the kidneys fail to function in a number of different ways (e.g. problems with salt/water homeostasis, BP control, removal of uraemic toxins, calcium/phosphate balance, potassium balance, acid-base balance). Depending on the underlying problem, these will result in peripheral/pulmonary oedema, hypertension, uraemia or metabolic acidosis.

Without transplantation, chronic renal failure can progress to end-stage renal failure (ESRF).

Diagnosis, screening and investigations
People with CRF may present with a range of signs and symptoms (e.g. shortness of breath, swollen ankles/feet/hands, tiredness, nausea, haematuria). CRF may have an insidious onset or present as a uraemic emergency. Screening for proteinuria helps to detect CRF in people at risk of its development (e.g. those with diabetes, hypertension, a family history of CRF or kidney injury). Renal ultrasound, biopsy and serum creatinine clearance may also aid in diagnosis.

Treatment
Treatment focuses on managing the presenting symptoms, aggressive blood pressure control to reduce the speed of deterioration and renal replacement therapy (dialysis/transplantation). There are two main dialysis options: haemodialysis and peritoneal dialysis. Haemodialysis involves the diffusion of solutes and water from blood across a semi-permeable membrane held in a haemodialysis machine. Filtered blood is returned to the circulatory system. Haemodialysis requires vascular access, preferably through an arteriovenous fistula. The fistula usually comprises a permanent anastomosis in the lower arm between the radial artery and the cephalic vein. Haemodialysis can result in cardiovascular instability.

Peritoneal dialysis (PD) is an alternative to haemodialysis. There are two types: continuous ambulatory peritoneal dialysis (CAPD) and automated peritoneal dialysis (APD). Both use the peritoneal lining as the dialysis membrane. CAPD requires patients to instil around 2 litres of isotonic or hypertonic glucose solution four times a day into the peritoneal cavity through a permanent catheter placed through the abdominal wall. Once instilled, the fluid is left in place for several (~6) hours and then, containing excess fluid, solutes and waste products, it is drained out. This needs to be done four times a day. Alternatively, the catheter is connected to a machine that does this overnight (APD). PD means that patients can be more independent of healthcare services once they are proficient in the technique. Dehydration, constipation and peritonitis are risks associated with PD. Dialysis requires patients to keep to strict dietary and fluid restrictions.

Renal transplantation is often the most effective treatment option.

Nursing care
The nursing care of patients with chronic renal failure depends largely on the stage of their disease and their treatment plan. However, restoring and maintaining homeostasis are central to care, as is helping the patient and family achieve the best quality of life possible within the constraints of CRF and its treatment. For those with ESRF, end-of-life care will be a central component. Chronic renal failure and the need for dialysis can be very frightening for the patient and their family/carers, so accurate, explanatory and empathic communication is essential. Self-management of CAPD at home relies on careful teaching and confidence building. Raising the possibility of kidney donation by relatives might be appropriate if transplantation is an option.

Cirrhosis
Definition
Cirrhosis is scarring of the liver, which in some people may lead to liver failure or cancer. Scarring occurs because as the liver recovers from inflammation (hepatitis), fibrous tissue and scars form. Cirrhosis reduces normal liver functioning and may result in chronic liver disease.

Some people with chronic liver disease may be relatively well (their condition is described as compensated), but others may be seriously ill (decompensated).

Chronic liver disease is associated with reduced liver cell mass and portal vein hypertension causing varices, ascites, encephalopathy (reversible) and jaundice. A patient's condition can deteriorate rapidly because of, for instance, GI bleeds, sepsis and electrolyte disturbance.

Diagnosis and investigations
Clinical examination, history taking, liver function and other blood tests, ultrasonography and biopsy.

Treatment
Depends on the extent and type of the cirrhosis.

Nursing care
Nursing care will focus on symptom control and management and should be tailored to the patient's needs while being alert to indications of deterioration (e.g. for encephalopathy – alterations to mood, attention span or consciousness and reversal of sleep patterns; for bleeding from GI tract – monitor vital signs; vomit and stool for blood). If ascites is present the patient may find mobilising difficult, be breathless and require a sodium-free diet and restricted fluid intake; as they are likely to be taking diuretics they will need easy access to a commode or toilet unless catheterised. If cirrhosis is due to alcohol dependency the patient may be anxious about stopping drinking and support and counselling will be needed; drugs will be prescribed to minimise symptoms of alcohol withdrawal. Ruptured varices may create torrential gastro-intestinal bleeding, which is a medical emergency.

Coagulation disorders
Definition
Disorders of coagulation affect clotting factors.

These disorders are categorised through routine coagulation tests: activated partial thromboplastin time (APTT), prothrombin time (PT) and thrombin time (TT).

Coagulation disorders can be inherited (e.g. haemophilia A, haemophilia B and von Willebrand's disease) or acquired (e.g. disseminated intravascular coagulation [DIC], liver disease and vitamin K deficiency).

Diagnosis and investigations
Coagulation tests: activated partial thromboplastin time (APTT), prothrombin time (PT) and thrombin time (TT).

Treatment
Depends on the underlying pathology.

Nursing care
Depends on the underlying pathology and signs, symptoms and treatments.

Constipation
Definition
Constipation is an alteration to normal bowel patterns characterised by infrequently passing hard, difficult-to-pass stools. These stools may be small or large. Constipation can be accompanied by abdominal pain, bloating and flatulence; and can be acute or chronic.

Constipation is commonly caused by diet (e.g. insufficient fibre and dehydration), lack of exercise and immobility, metabolic disorders (e.g. diabetes mellitus, uraemia), obstruction (e.g. megacolon, cancer, anal fissures), neuropathies (e.g. Parkinson's disease, multiple sclerosis), bowel disease (e.g. irritable bowel syndrome) or depression.

Diarrhoea can accompany constipation and often manifests as faecal incontinence. In this case more fluid stool passes around the obstruction caused by the impacted stool.

Diagnosis
History and clinical examination.

Treatment
Depends on the underlying cause.

Nursing care
Find out about the current episode of constipation and whether or not constipation is a common feature in the patient's life. Ask about any possible triggers and ways of relieving constipation that the patient might have used.

Constipation can often be relieved by reviewing and altering drug regimens (refer to doctor), diet and exercise. Dietary alteration centres on increasing the amount of fibre in the diet and reducing refined products. Increasing physical exercise increases peristalsis and may reduce constipation. Dehydration may be linked to constipation, so increasing the amount of fluids consumed in a day may help (around ~2 litres is the usual daily intake).

Introducing more time for defecation during the day may be useful – many people simply do not allow enough time or ignore the urge to defecate. Thinking more about the position used for defecating might also be helpful. Crouching is the best position, so to mimic this sitting on the toilet with knees raised slightly by using a footstool may be helpful.

Laxatives may be suggested, starting with the lowest dose. Once constipation resolves then laxatives should be stopped. Sometimes enemas/suppositories are needed to manage chronic constipation. These should be administered in line with the manufacturer's recommendations and local policy.

Coronary heart disease
Definition
Coronary heart disease (CHD) is a collective name for diseases affecting the health of the heart muscle.

The coronary arteries provide the heart with important nutrients and oxygen to enable effective pumping. CHD is linked to coronary atherosclerosis (narrowing of the blood vessels' lumen due to the accumulation of atheroma) and resultant ischaemia or infarction. If a piece of atheroma breaks away from the artery wall, a blood clot forms around it, leading to blockage of a coronary artery. This causes damage to the myocardium, as nutrients and oxygen cannot reach the heart muscle.

Having CHD can increase your chances of having a heart attack (myocardial infarction, MI).

Angina and MI are the most common presentations of symptomatic CHD, which can be described as a spectrum with stable angina (exertional) at the less severe end and MI at the most severe. Unstable angina and heart attacks are also referred to as acute coronary syndrome (ACS).

CHD is a significant cause of death in men and women.

Risk factors

- High blood pressure
- High blood cholesterol levels
- Family history of CHD
- Smoking
- Physical inactivity
- Being overweight
- Poor diet – high in fat and low in fibre
- Excessive alcohol consumption
- Diabetes.

Diagnosis and investigations
History and clinical examination; ECG; exercise tolerance tests; blood tests (e.g. cholesterol testing, cardiac enzyme tests); echocardiogram, cardiac angiogram and other imaging techniques.

Treatment
Depends on presenting symptoms and diagnosis.

Nursing care
Providing the right nursing care for people with CHD depends on the severity of their presenting symptoms and their diagnosis. Nursing is likely to be mainly associated with giving advice about diet, lifestyle (alcohol and smoking), exercise and medication.

Crohn's disease
Definition
Crohn's disease (CD) is a chronic inflammatory disease affecting any part of the GI tract, from the mouth to the anus. Inflammation in CD is not contiguous as it is in ulcerative colitis (UC). A characteristic pattern of affected and unaffected portions is present: 'skip' lesions. Ulcers are deeper than in UC and sometimes lead to fistulae and abscesses. Symptoms depend on the location. CD often presents with abdominal pain, malaise and diarrhoea. It is incurable, characterised by remissions and relapses, associated with high morbidity and can result in reduced life expectancy. Extra-intestinal problems include ankylosing spondylitis and uveitis.

Diagnosis and investigations
History and clinical examination. Stool samples may be taken to rule out other problems. Colonoscopy/endoscopy may be performed, as may other imaging tests.

Treatment
Treatment is by medication and surgery when complications (e.g. fistulae, abscesses) occur. Nutritional assessment and support are also essential components of treatment.

Nursing care
People with CD often require nursing in hospital. Hospitalisation focuses on intravenous medication, fluid replacement, nutritional support and/or surgery. People admitted to hospital will often be debilitated and anxious. Over half of those with CD will require surgery and this will cause anxiety, associated with the possibility of stoma formation and management.

Dementias

Definition

Dementia is a global impairment of cognition with normal levels of consciousness. (N.B. By contrast, in acute confusional states consciousness is impaired.) Dementia is generally a disease of old age. The more common types are Alzheimer's disease, vascular dementia, dementia with Lewy bodies (DLB) and frontotemporal dementia (FTD).

Younger people may have dementia due to HIV (human immunodeficiency virus), vasculitis, new-variant CJD (Creutzfeldt–Jakob disease) or end-stage multiple sclerosis.

It is sometimes hard to determine the specific type of dementia that affects people, so it is wise to focus on the impact of the dementia and how nursing care can best be used to improve the quality of life, not only of the person with dementia but also of their family and carers.

Having dementia will result in increased dependence on others to maintain activities of daily living.

For the majority of people with dementia, deterioration in memory and thinking abilities will also eventually be accompanied by physical decline (e.g. incontinence of urine and faeces).

Diagnosis and investigations

The early stages of dementia can be hard to detect reliably, so referral to the GP or memory clinic is important.

Specialist memory and cognitive tests, history and CT brain scans may be taken.

Treatment

Dementia cannot be cured and is a progressive disease; progress can be slowed in some people by early treatment, for example the use of Aricept for people with Alzheimer's disease. Providing the best care for someone with dementia will require the efforts of the entire multi-disciplinary team, since attention will need to be given to the physical, environmental, social, emotional and psychological aspects of care. Family and carers will also need high levels of support and advice. Balancing the needs of the family/carers with the needs of the person with dementia is sometimes complex and challenging.

Dementia will progress differently in different people, so it is important to care for each person as an individual and to address each of their difficulties as it occurs.

Nursing care

The goal of nursing is to achieve person-centred care delivered in a safe environment. People with dementia may feel isolated and disorientated; they will easily forget why they are there, what they have been asked to do and who you are, so ensuring a consistent approach to care from all nurses is important. Repeated gentle reminders about who you are and the treatments/care you are proposing are important ways to increase a person's compliance with care and also their feelings of safety and security.

All nurses will provide care to people with dementia, either focusing specifically on dementia care or on other acute illnesses or disorders experienced by a person with dementia. As dementia is a progressive disease, and is naturally associated with the later stages of life, nurses providing palliative and end-of-life care will also become involved.

Some nurses specialise in dementia care (e.g. those working in community mental health teams and Admiral Nurses working alongside Dementia UK). Many wards in acute hospitals will have a nurse identified as a dementia champion too; these nurses have specialist knowledge of the needs of people with dementia.

Diabetes mellitus
Definition
Diabetes mellitus is a disease characterised by raised blood glucose levels. In people with diabetes a random test for blood glucose will show an elevated blood glucose level of >11.1 mmol/L. In diabetes glucagon raises blood glucose levels too much, because either there is no insulin to inhibit it or the body has become resistant to the effects of insulin.

Diabetes mellitus can take two forms: Type 1 diabetes (a relatively rare condition) and Type 2 diabetes (which is becoming increasingly common). Type 1 diabetes is associated with a total lack of/deficiency in insulin because of pancreatic islet beta cell deficiency. This may have an autoimmune origin. Type 2 diabetes is associated with insulin resistance rather than deficiency. In this type of diabetes the body's cells become resistant to the effects of insulin and require more to keep blood glucose levels within normal limits. Type 2 diabetes is usually linked to being overweight.

Type 1 diabetes tends to present in people aged below 30, whereas Type 2 diabetes presents in people aged around 50 or over. Type 2 diabetes is common in South Asian and African Caribbean people.

Some pregnant women can get gestational diabetes and require specialist care. They may have a risk of developing Type 2 diabetes later.

Symptoms of diabetes include increased thirst, increased urine output, tiredness and weight loss. Diabetes is linked to long-term complications (e.g. kidney damage, foot ulceration, poor wound healing, retinal damage and sight deterioration).

Diagnosis and investigations
Diagnosis and monitoring of people with diabetes involves testing the blood for blood glucose level and for HbA1c (glycated haemoglobin), a measure of average blood glucose over a few weeks or months. Urinalysis will also show glucose. A glucose tolerance test (GTT) can be administered.

Treatment
Treatment is with injected insulin replacement in people with Type 1 diabetes and with diet, lifestyle changes and oral drugs to reduce hyperglycaemia in people with Type 2 diabetes.

Nursing care
Nurses will care for people with either type of diabetes mellitus, but there are differences in the care associated with each type.

For people with Type 1 diabetes, regular injections of insulin, careful attention to diet and close self-monitoring of blood glucose levels will enable them to maintain blood glucose levels within normal limits. People are usually diagnosed with Type 1 diabetes in childhood or adolescence, and so by the time adulthood is reached they are skilled at controlling their diabetes effectively. However, extra stresses placed on the body by, for instance, infection, trauma, surgery, inadequate attention to diet or failure to use insulin correctly may necessitate a reappraisal of their condition and intervention by specialist diabetes nurses or practice nurses. Some people may develop diabetic ketoacidosis (DKA) as a result of severe hyperglycaemia and be admitted to hospital; they will require close monitoring of vital signs and level of consciousness, rehydration, electrolyte balance restoration and insulin therapy. Any underlying infection will also need treating, which may necessitate the administration of antibiotics or other medications. Ongoing monitoring of people with Type 1 diabetes is likely to be undertaken by practice nurses.

For the majority of people with Type 2 diabetes, their nursing care will be provided by practice nurses and/or community nurses. This care will focus initially around accurate assessment and regular monitoring of their diabetes, combined with education about medication, the risks associated with diabetes and the possible requirement to alter diet and exercise patterns, as well as to be aware that extra care needs to be taken of feet, heart and eye health.

Diarrhoea
Definition
Diarrhoea is characterised by the frequent passing of loose/watery stools. It can be accompanied by abdominal pain, bloating and flatulence. Diarrhoea is commonly caused by diet (e.g. excess ingestion of bran/fibre supplements, allergies and food intolerances), infections, medications (e.g. antibiotics, antihypertensive drugs), bowel diseases (irritable bowel syndrome, inflammatory bowel disease) and anxiety.

Diarrhoea can be acute or chronic. It can accompany constipation and often manifests as faecal incontinence. In this case more fluid stool passes around the obstruction caused by the impacted stool.

Diagnosis
History taking and if necessary stool specimen or other investigations.

Treatment
Dependent on cause. Rehydration and if needed anti-diarrhoeal drugs.

Nursing care
Find out more about the current episode of diarrhoea. Ask about any possible triggers and ways of relieving diarrhoea that the patient might have used.

If in hospital, try to make sure the patient is close to a toilet or has a commode within the bed space. Ensure that curtains are easily closable and can be securely fastened.

Acute diarrhoea is often mild and self-limiting and care is given in the community. Advice should be given about hydration and the use of anti-diarrhoeal over-the-counter drugs (e.g. loperamide) and/or rehydration medication (e.g. dioralyte).

If infective diarrhoea is suspected, advice about infection control and hand washing should be given.

Chronic diarrhoea needs to be managed in relation to the underlying cause. Some anti-diarrhoeal drugs may be prescribed.

Discuss lifestyle modifications if appropriate, such as dietary modifications.

Diverticular disease
Definition
Diverticular disease is a degenerative change in the colon that causes the formation of out-pouches or pockets of mucosa that push through the muscular wall of the bowel and form a diverticulum. Symptoms include constipation, intermittent constipation with intermittent diarrhoea, and spasmodic grumbling-type pain. The colon may become inflamed as a result of impaction of faeces in a diverticulum, which in turn can result in infection and abscess formation, pain and fever. This is known as diverticulitis. The diverticulum can erode blood vessels, resulting in GI tract bleeding, or form fistulae with neighbouring organs; it may also perforate, causing peritonitis. Diverticular disease is more common in older people, but is often asymptomatic.

Diagnosis and investigations
History and CT imaging, colonoscopy.

Treatment
Treatment depends on the presenting problem, but is generally conservative (e.g. avoiding constipation by dietary modification, intravenous fluids and anti-spasmodic medication), although surgery may be needed.

Nursing care
The routine nursing care of people with diverticular disease focuses on health education and promotion as well as symptom control and management, and is predominantly about giving dietary advice. Anti-spasmodic medication may be prescribed. Patients should be told to avoid stimulant laxatives, since increasing the pressure on the colon's muscular wall can cause the development of more diverticula. Hospitalisation may be necessary if pain is severe, dehydration occurs or there is infection. Surgery may also be necessary. As with other inflammatory intestinal conditions, fear of stoma formation may be present.

Eczema
Definition
Eczema is an inflammation of the skin. Its severity can range from mild to severe.
Eczema typically presents with reddened, itchy, scaly patches, which may be on the face
or in the body's flexures. Scratching may cause infections.
Eczema tends to flare up from time to time, sometimes in response to known triggers.
It cannot be cured, but patients can manage it very successfully through the use of
emollients, atopic corticosteroid treatments, oral antihistamines and avoiding triggers.
Severe eczema can result in the need for hospitalisation, especially if skin failure or
infection occurs.

Diagnosis and investigations
History and clinical examination.

Treatment
Includes the use of emollients, atopic corticosteroid treatments, oral antihistamines and
avoiding triggers (e.g. some foodstuffs, animal fur, certain cosmetic preparations or stress).

Nursing care
Eczema is usually managed in the community, so practice nurses are likely to have a large
part to play in health education and promotion as well as symptom control and management.
Specialist dermatological nurses will also be involved, although their involvement may be
associated more with severe eczema. Occupational health nurses will be involved in
care if eczema is work related (either through contact with irritants or as a result of
work-related stress).

Encephalitis
Definition
Encephalitis is a serious, potentially fatal infection of the brain requiring prompt diagnosis, treatment and hospitalisation. It may also leave people functionally and intellectually impaired – sometimes to the extent that they require long-term ongoing care.
Encephalitis can have a rapid onset.
Immunisation is available against some types of encephalitis.

Diagnosis and investigations
Physical examination, history taking, blood tests and culture, lumbar puncture, CT and MRI scans.

Treatment
Depends on presentation and likely infective agent.

Nursing care
Nursing care will largely focus on making regular neurological assessments and reporting alterations. It is important to be alert for signs of raised intracranial pressure (raised blood pressure, slowed pulse and altered/irregular respirations) and to report these immediately. It is also important to assess, treat and monitor pain (e.g. headaches) and nausea/vomiting.
Assess the patient's ability to engage in activities of daily living and alter care accordingly.

Endocrine disorders
Definition
The endocrine system contributes to maintaining homeostasis, coordinating the body's storage and use of carbohydrates, proteins and fats for energy, regulating growth, metabolism, ions (e.g. sodium, potassium and calcium) and reproduction, and responding to external stimuli (e.g. temperature and stress). The endocrine system does this by producing hormones.

This system comprises three parts:

- Endocrine glands (organs whose sole function is to produce hormones – pituitary, thyroid, parathyroid and adrenal glands).
- Organs that produce large amounts of hormones but have other functions (hypothalamus and pancreas).
- Hormone-producing cells in organs that have many other functions other than producing hormones (e.g. stomach, small intestines, ovaries, testes).

Each part of the endocrine system is served by a rich blood supply, enabling hormones to be easily transported around the body.

The endocrine system's influence extends throughout the body, so failure in any part of it can have significant consequences for a person's health. Disorders of the endocrine system include diabetes mellitus, hypo/hyperthyroidism, adrenal disease, diabetes insipidus, acromegaly, prolactin hypersecretion, hyper/hypocalcaemia and hypogonadism.

End-of-life care
Definition
End-of-life care focuses attention on the palliation (easing) of symptoms associated with the process of dying. These are largely pain, alterations to breathing and restlessness or distress.

Nurses need to focus on the person who is dying and their family and friends, who may be made anxious and distressed by these symptoms, thereby increasing their own feelings of anxiety, uncertainty and imminent loss. Nursing care needs to focus also on the environment. Death can occur in many places: some people will die at home, in a care home or residential home or in a hospice; others will die in hospital, in the ward, the ED or a side room. Whichever it is, nurses should if possible create a private, comfortable area and stay with the patient (and their family if they wish).

Excellent nursing care at the end of life is a balance of technical competence to ease symptoms; the promotion/facilitation of appropriate physical, emotional, cultural and spiritual comfort; and skilled communication to reduce anxiety by explanations, listening and 'being there' to create (if possible) an environment within which intense and mixed emotions can be felt and expressed.

During and after death there may be particular wishes or customs that the dying person and their family/friends would want to be performed. Nurses need to know what these are and to help facilitate them if possible.

After death there are several formalities that need to be undertaken (e.g. certification of death by a doctor, arranging for the person's body to be removed). Using the gap between death and the finalisation of these aspects of care to allow relatives to be alone with the patient's body may be helpful for them – ask them if they would like this. Remember, though, that if they do want this you should arrange to come back in a short time to see how they are. Some people will want to be by themselves in these circumstances and a quiet, comfortable room close at hand should be found. Tea and coffee will usually be appreciated at this time too.

The family/friends may want to assist with laying the person out (last offices) and you should ask if they would like to help you do this. Some people may prefer to stay and watch rather than help; others will prefer to leave and come back later. For some people being able to join you at this final stage of care may be a comforting act of farewell.

Nurses rarely 'get used' to death; you and your colleagues may continue to find death distressing throughout your career, especially if it is unexpected or you have known the patient for a long time. It is important to take a little time for yourself after a patient's death, even if it is only a short break on the ward.

Epilepsy
Definition
Epilepsy is an intense burst of electrical activity in the brain that causes a temporary disruption to the way the brain normally works; this means that the brain's messages get 'mixed up' (Epilepsy Action, https://www.epilepsy.org.uk/campaigns/epilepsy-week/2013/seizures-look-the-same) and alterations occur to motor, sensory or psychological functions. The disordered electrical discharge can happen in different parts of the brain, so epilepsy manifests in different ways.

Sudden-onset epilepsy can also be the first indication of another central nervous system (CNS) disorder, such as a space-occupying lesion. New seizures should always be investigated thoroughly.

When epilepsy is poorly controlled, either through poor drug compliance or for instance hypoglycaemia or alcohol withdrawal, seizures can happen continuously (status epilepticus). They may occur one after another or a seizure may appear to last longer than normal. Status epilepticus is a very serious condition requiring immediate medical intervention. Untreated status epilepticus has high morbidity and mortality due to cerebral oedema and cardiorespiratory arrest.

Diagnosis and investigations
History taking from the patient and reliable observers. Electroencephalographs (EEG) and brain imaging.

Treatment
Epilepsy is an ongoing condition that is controlled by medication. Successful management of epilepsy rather than cure is the objective of care. Some people experience side effects due to their medication and so for this reason (and sometimes others) compliance with medication can be poor. Medication for epilepsy can also interact with other medications (e.g. oral contraceptives) and therefore discussion of the range of medications taken is important.

Nursing care
People living with epilepsy and their family/carers will require routine support and education from practice nurses, occupational health nurses and nurses working in the ED or acute wards (if their epilepsy is not well controlled by medication). Family planning nurses may also be involved in discussions about contraceptive effectiveness and pre-conceptual care with women of child-bearing age.

Status epilepticus is a medical emergency requiring immediate attention. Medical care largely focuses on terminating the seizures, for example with IV diazepam or anti-epileptics, and maintaining the airway and cardiac output.

Fractures
Definition
A fracture occurs when an abnormal force is exerted on a normal bone or a moderate force on a diseased bone (e.g. one with metastases or osteoporosis).
Fractures can be:

- Simple (a clean break with no protrusion through the skin).
- Compound (a break through the skin).
- Complicated (another structure involved, e.g. nerve, blood vessel).
- Comminuted (more than two fragments of bone).
- Greenstick (incomplete).
- Pathological (bone weakened by disease).

Fracture repair may be complicated by blood loss, infection, fat embolism following fracture/cutting of long bones, venous thromboembolism (VTE), compartment syndrome (bleeding/swelling within a tightly enclosed space, e.g. a bundle of tightly confined muscle fibres; acute signs and symptoms include intense pain, pins and needles/tingling/burning sensations on skin, paralysis, pallor and lack of pulse), poor union of bones or arthritis.
Compartment syndrome is an emergency.

Diagnosis and investigations
Examination, history and imaging.

Treatment
Depends on type and location of fracture.

Nursing care
Nurses will work with people with fractures in the ED, in the community (e.g. immediately following a fall or after discharge from hospital) and in hospital wards and specialist orthopaedic units.
A person with a fracture will require immediate pain relief, reassurance and explanation about investigations (X-rays) and treatment (e.g. methods of reduction and immobilisation, their likely length of stay, whether or not they will have a plaster cast). They will need help with their usual activities of daily living and maintaining dignity whether they are in hospital or at home.

Gallstone disease

Definition
Gallstone disease can affect the gall bladder; the gall bladder and the common bile duct; or the pancreas. Gallstones contain cholesterol or bile pigments or both mixed together. Gallstones can obstruct the bile duct and may be present in the gall bladder (cholelithiasis). They can be asymptomatic or symptomatic.

Gallstone disease is more common in women than in men.

The location of the obstruction determines signs, symptoms and treatment. Signs and symptoms include pain (sudden and severe or grumbling) in the right upper quadrant of the abdomen (often brought on by fatty food); nausea, vomiting; fever if infection; obstructive jaundice (cholestatic jaundice) with pale stools and orange urine (biliary obstruction).

Gallstones are a major cause of pancreatitis, when stones move down the common bile duct and through the hepatopancreatic ampulla. Gallstones frequently accompany cancer of the gall bladder. If gallstones pass into the small intestine, this may cause intestinal obstruction (gallstone ileus).

Diagnosis and investigations
History, examination, ultrasonography and endoscopic retrograde cholangiopancreatography (ERCP).

Treatment
Active monitoring if asymptomatic; lifestyle changes may control initial episodes of biliary colic (reduced fatty diet and small, frequent meals); IV antibiotics to treat infection; ERCP to remove stones in the common bile duct; open, keyhole or laparoscopic surgical removal of the gall bladder (cholecystectomy; emergency, planned following treatment for cholecystitis, or elective following periods of biliary colic and confirmed gallstones).

Nursing care
If a cholecystectomy is required nursing care will focus on the principles of pre- and post-operative care. Length of time in hospital will depend on the operation performed and any pre-/post-operative complications (e.g. infection).

Gastritis
Definition
Gastritis is an acute or chronic inflammation of the lining of the stomach. Acute gastritis can be caused by ingestion of irritants (e.g. aspirin, alcohol) or by bacteria (helicobacter pylori). Helicobacter pylori is a common cause of chronic gastritis.

Pain (before or after food), nausea and vomiting are common symptoms associated with acute gastritis. Rarely patients experience haematemesis, melaena, weight loss or iron-deficiency anaemia. Occult blood may be present in faeces.

Patients with pernicious anaemia, autoimmune disorders, chronic alcoholism, long-term use of NSAIDs (non-steroidal anti-inflammatory drugs) and peptic ulcers may have chronic gastritis. Most people with gastritis are cared for at home by their GP. Practice nurses may provide advice for patients with gastritis about diet (e.g. avoiding spicy foods and alcohol) and medication.

Diagnosis and investigations
Endoscopy and gastric biopsy. Blood and breath tests are also available for detecting helicobacter pylori.

Treatment
Dietary alteration and medication.

Nursing care
The nursing care of patients with gastritis focuses on health education and health promotion. Encouraging patients to alter their diet to avoid spicy food, alcohol and any other identifiable triggers is important. The importance of avoiding aspirin and over-the-counter NSAIDs should also be emphasised. Patients should be reminded to seek urgent medical advice if symptoms worsen or if new signs and symptoms appear (e.g. haematemesis, melaena, weight loss or tiredness).

Gastroenteritis
Definition
Gastroenteritis is an infection of the intestines most commonly caused by viruses or bacteria. Acute gastroenteritis typically presents as diarrhoea with or without vomiting and is accompanied by abdominal pain, pyrexia, headache and myalgia. Onset is usually sudden and most cases of acute gastroenteritis settle with little intervention. Patients are treated in primary care and advised about hydration, rehydration medication (e.g. dioralyte) and cross-infection. If symptoms persist, a stool specimen should be sent for analysis so that treatment can be tailored to the cause. Antibiotics may be prescribed against bacterial gastroenteritis if symptoms persist. Viral infections include those from noroviruses and are easily spread through contact with unwashed hands and/or surfaces.

Patients needing hospitalisation are likely to be older, dehydrated, exhausted or have an infection caused by a more serious causative agent (e.g. *E. Coli* O157 or *clostridium botulinum*). Intravenous fluids and antibiotics may be needed.

Chronic gastroenteritis may be caused by giardiasis, gastro-intestinal tuberculosis or amoebas. Treatment is usually with medication. Attention should be drawn to rehydration.

Diagnosis and investigations
History and stool specimen.

Treatment
Depends on cause, but rehydration is always important.

Nursing care
The nursing care of people with gastro-intestinal infections, whether in primary care or in hospitals, focuses on rehydration, symptom control and infection control.

Gastro-oesophageal reflux disease
Definition
Gastro-oesophageal reflux disease (GORD) commonly presents with heartburn, effortless regurgitation, belching and sometimes nausea. These symptoms can be linked to particular positions, such as bending forwards or lying down. Intermittent pain on swallowing may also be present. Chest pain may occur, so angina needs to be ruled out before a diagnosis of GORD can be made.

Lifestyle factors including smoking, obesity, stress, fatty foods, pastry, alcohol and chocolate can exacerbate symptoms.

Diagnosis and investigations
History, upper gastro-intestinal endoscopy and, if symptoms persist, manometry and pH recording.

Treatment
Management is primarily through lifestyle changes and medication, for example antacids, proton pump inhibitors (PPIs), prokinetics or H2-receptor antagonists (H2RAs); surgery may be necessary for those with hiatus hernias, such as laparoscopic anti-reflux surgery (LARS).

Nursing care
Depends on treatment but is likely to focus on supporting lifestyle changes. If surgery is required care will focus on the principles of pre- and post-operative care. Special preparation may be needed for some procedures and these may vary according to local practice.

Glaucoma

Definition

Glaucoma causes damage to the optic nerve because of increased intra-ocular pressure. Glaucoma may occur at any age, but is more common after the age of 40 years. Glaucoma may be acute or chronic. In chronic glaucoma symptoms are usually noticed when peripheral vision lessens (becomes tunnel-like).

Diagnosis and investigations

Eye examination and intra-ocular pressure measurement.

Treatment

The aim of treatment in both acute and chronic glaucoma is to reduce damage (repair of already acquired loss of vision is not possible in chronic glaucoma); options include eye drops to lower intra-ocular pressure by reducing the amount of aqueous fluid produced and increasing the opening of the drainage channels in the eye. Laser surgery, performed under local anaesthetic as a day case/outpatient, may also be used to improve drainage.

Nursing care

Nursing care for people with glaucoma will focus on teaching eye drop use and monitoring compliance (in some instances, for instance if manual dexterity is compromised, drops will need to be administered). If surgery is performed, care will focus also on information giving and reassurance.

Glomerulonephritis
Definition
Glomerulonephritis (GN) means inflammation of the glomeruli and is characterised by the presence of protein, blood and casts (cylindrical structures formed in the nephrons) in urine.

GN accounts for renal failure in around one-third of patients needing renal dialysis or renal transplant. It affects both kidneys symmetrically and can be acute or chronic. GN is also associated with systemic lupus erythematosus (SLE).

Diagnosis and investigations
Urinalysis and microscopy, 24-hour urine collection for protein excretion, serum creatinine and creatinine clearance, and renal ultrasound to establish the size of the kidneys. If the kidneys are normal in size, biopsies may be taken.

Treatment
GN is usually classified into three types:

• Minimal change GN (corticosteroid therapy to produce remission).
• Membranous GN (requires drug therapy and has a mixed prognosis).
• Rapidly progressive GN (requires aggressive drug therapy).

Raised blood pressure and raised cholesterol can result from GN. Aggressive drug therapy for both may slow the progress of the disease.

Nursing care
The nursing care of patients with glomerulonephritis will depend on the severity of the disease and may range from advice about diet and medication to supervision of home or hospital dialysis.

Gout
Definition
Gout is a crystal-related joint disorder in which crystals of monosodium urate accumulate in joints and result in synovitis (inflammation of the synovial membrane).

Joint pain, usually in one joint (monoarthritis; often the big toe), occurs with swelling, tenderness and redness in the surrounding tissues.

Acute gout may progress to chronic gout exacerbated by exercise, excessive alcohol or a diet high in purines. Uric acid crystals can form tophi on fingers or ear cartilage.

Gout is more common in men than in women and can be genetic.

Diagnosis and investigations
History, examination and blood tests (serum uric acid).

Treatment
Pain relief with non-steroidal anti-inflammatory drugs, uric acid–lowering medication and lifestyle/dietary modification.

Nursing care
Support with lifestyle modification.

Haemorrhoids
Definition
Haemorrhoids (piles) are submucosal vascular structures consisting of a dilated venous plexus, a small artery and areolar tissue in the anal canal. Swollen piles result from increased venous pressure from straining to defecate or altered haemodynamics, for instance during pregnancy. They can be itchy and may bleed or prolapse.

Diagnosis
History and examination.

Treatment
Treatment in the first instance consists of using bulk laxatives and eating a high-fibre diet to prevent constipation and straining. Injection sclerotherapy, cryosurgery or haemorrhoidectomy may be necessary if bleeding or prolapse occurs.

Nursing care
Nursing will focus on giving dietary advice (increased fibre, increased fluid intake and increased exercise) to minimise constipation and associated straining and/or pre- and post-operative care if surgery is needed (this is likely to be undertaken as a day case). Reassurance and prophylactic pain control will be needed post-operatively around the time of the patient's first post-surgery bowel opening.

Hearing loss
Definition
Hearing loss in adults may be congenital or acquired, for example as a result of trauma (e.g. excess noise, head injury), illness (e.g. Ménière's disease) or ageing. There are two categories of hearing loss: conductive and sensorineural. Acute hearing loss may be caused by foreign bodies or an accumulation of wax in the external auditory canal or infection (e.g. otitis media). These sorts of problems prevent sound waves passing through to the cochlear (conduction deafness). Conductive hearing loss may be alleviated by removal of wax or foreign bodies or the treatment of infection with antibiotics, if appropriate. Sensorineural deafness (e.g. age-related hearing loss, congenital malformations, Ménière's disease) is likely to be a result of a defect in the cochlea or its connecting nerve.

Age-related hearing loss (presbycusis) is characterised by an inability to hear both high and low frequencies. Many people experience natural age-related changes to their hearing as they grow older, so it is particularly important that if older people (or their family/friends) notice a hearing loss, they are assessed and treated quickly.

Diagnosis and investigations
History, examination and hearing tests.

Treatment
Treatment is dependent on cause. If hearing loss is confirmed, regular review by an audiologist is important to ensure that the best hearing possible is achieved using aids and other hearing technologies.

Nursing care
Hearing loss can result in isolation, frustration and depression, so sensitive and appropriate education, reassurance, referral for aids (e.g. hearing aids or amplified, vibrating and flashing phones/alarms) and monitoring of the use and effectiveness of any hearing aids should form the foundation of skilled nursing care for people with a hearing loss. Nursing someone with hearing loss can occur anywhere in the health and social care system. Clear communication and use of hearing aids where worn are essential.

Heart failure
Definition
Heart failure (HF) is a serious, potentially fatal, clinical syndrome that has impacts on multiple systems, resulting from the inability to maintain adequate cardiac output.

HF can be acute or chronic. Acute HF is a sudden loss of cardiac function, for example secondary to ACS, causing pulmonary oedema and cardiogenic shock. Chronic heart failure (CHF) is complex and progressive, and is due to insufficient cardiac output to meet the demands of the body. Chronic heart failure is a common problem for older people, accounting for at least 5% of admissions to medical and elderly care wards.

A common cause of HF is impaired ventricular contraction, for instance due to damaged myocardium. HF can involve either ventricle by itself or both. Left heart failure (LHF) results in the build-up of blood returning from the lungs in the left ventricle and atrium and congestion of the lungs. This causes breathlessness (which worsens when lying down), fatigue and an enlarged heart. Right heart failure (RHF) means that de-oxygenated blood from the body (systemic) cannot efficiently be pumped to the lungs. This causes congestion in the systemic circulatory system, resulting in fluid retention in the legs (oedema) and, if severe, ascites. RHF may occur because of lung problems, embolism or valve disease, but is most likely because of the presence of LHF.

People living with heart failure are likely to visit their GP frequently, so much of the care is provided in primary care.

Diagnosis and investigations
Examination, history, echocardiogram, ECG and chest X-ray.

Treatment
Treat underlying cause and any arrhythmias. Consider dietary restrictions.

Medication including diuretics, ACE (angiotensin-converting enzyme) inhibitors, angiotensin II receptor antagonists and digoxin.

Nursing care
Nursing largely focuses on the management of medications and addressing symptoms in line with the patient's wishes. Although people may be admitted to hospital with varying degrees of heart failure, much of the care for those with HF is undertaken in primary care. Nurses may need to help people deal with symptoms such as breathlessness, anorexia, oedema (ankle and sacrum), disorientation, fatigue, poor wound healing and risk of pressure ulcers, diminished urinary output, cyanosis and cold feet and hands.

Hepatitis
Definition
Hepatitis is inflammation of the liver. It can be acute or chronic. Acute hepatitis is caused by viruses or reactions to drugs/toxins or, rarely, an autoimmune response. Chronic hepatitis is when symptoms of acute hepatitis remain or liver function tests continue to be abnormal six months after the initial onset of the illness.

Hepatitis is sometimes referred to as viral hepatitis and non-viral hepatitis. Viruses cause hepatitis A, B, C, D and E. Non-viral hepatitis is due to drug reactions (drug-induced hepatitis), excessive alcohol consumption (alcohol-induced hepatitis) or autoimmune response (autoimmune hepatitis).

Viral hepatitis is usually self-limiting with a good prognosis. The signs and symptoms of viral hepatitis are initial flu-like symptoms (e.g. headache, fever, nasal congestion, sore throat, mild upper abdominal pain and nausea and vomiting), followed by jaundice due to raised bilirubin levels in the blood and the depositing of bile pigments in sclera, skin and mucous membranes. Urine may be orange in colour and stools white due to intrahepatic cholestasis. Jaundice typically resolves in about two weeks with complete recovery. Liver enzymes will be raised.

Drug-induced hepatitis can result from several drugs. Taking an overdose of paracetamol is a common cause and rapid (<8 hours after ingestion) intravenous administration of an antidote should be given to prevent fatal liver failure.

In alcohol-induced hepatitis the signs and symptoms are lethargy, diarrhoea, vomiting, malnourishment, malaise, pain in the upper abdomen, fever, an enlarged liver and jaundice.

Chronic hepatitis is usually associated with hepatitis B, C or D, autoimmune hepatitis and alcohol- or drug-related disease. Chronic hepatitis may lead to scarring of the liver (cirrhosis), which in some people leads to liver failure or cancer. Scarring occurs because as the liver recovers from inflammation fibrous tissue and scars form. Cirrhosis reduces normal liver functioning.

Diagnosis and investigations
Examination, history, liver function and other blood tests, ultrasonography and biopsy.

Treatment
Depends on cause and symptoms.

Nursing care
Acute viral hepatitis, without complications, requires little nursing intervention except for advice from the practice nurse about how to deal with symptoms (e.g. rest, eat an easily digested light diet of small, high-calorie meals and drink extra fluids if feverish). An alternative to paracetamol to reduce pain and pyrexia should be sought; paracetamol should only be taken at doses prescribed by the GP. Patients should be reminded to seek medical advice if their symptoms persist for longer than 3–4 weeks, if symptoms worsen or if new signs and symptoms appear (e.g. confusion, altered mood, drowsiness, fits). Advice should also be given about minimising the spread of infection – close contacts (people the person lives with/cooks for/has sex with) should be advised to see their GP, since early vaccination may prevent the disease developing in them. Sometimes people with acute hepatitis require hospitalisation and in these cases nursing care will focus on the presenting signs and symptoms.

HIV
Definition
Human immunodeficiency virus (HIV) is a retrovirus that infects T-helper cells, compromising their surface protein CD4 and macrophages. Gradually the immune system becomes seriously affected and susceptible to many different types of infection and, rarely, cancers (e.g. non-Hodgkin's lymphoma or Kaposi's sarcoma). The blood-borne virus can be transmitted in a variety of ways (e.g. through sexual intercourse, contaminated blood products, needle-stick injuries or intravenous drug abuse, and through maternal–child transmission).

HIV tends to be asymptomatic after initial infection and this period without signs and symptoms can last for several years. During this time the virus can still be highly infectious. HIV may then progress to being symptomatic. It is classified as acquired immunodeficiency syndrome (AIDS) when the person has an AIDS-defining illness (e.g. oesophageal candidiasis, tuberculosis, lymphoma, recurrent herpes zooster).

People living with AIDS may have many debilitating problems, some of which nurses can help with, such as fever or breathlessness due to pneumonia or Kaposi's sarcoma. Symptom control and management are very important. Some people with AIDS will be severely ill (e.g. those with cerebral infections or AIDS-related dementia) or reaching the end of their lives; they will require appropriate care.

Health education about the spread of HIV/AIDS is essential in minimising the transmission of the virus through advice about safe sex through condom use, safer IV drug use by proper disposal of needles and never sharing them, and using reputable tattoo parlours.

Diagnosis and investigations
History and detection of anti-HIV antibodies.

Treatment
Treatment of HIV is usually through combinations of drugs, for instance highly active anti-retroviral therapy (HAART), and treatment of opportunistic infections. Better treatment over the last few years means that HIV is a less severe disease than first anticipated.

Nursing care
People with HIV/AIDS are usually linked to a specialist nurse who will advise them about the progress of their illness and how to maintain their health. For people with HIV advice about adhering to drug regimens, knowing the warning signs of deterioration, seeking advice about infections early and the need for protected sexual activity will be the mainstays of health education and health promotion.

Hypertension
Definition
Hypertension is when blood pressure is sustained at a level higher than 140/90 mmHg. Hypertension can be divided into essential (primarily associated with genetic and lifestyle factors but no single known cause) and secondary hypertension (due to other identifiable causes, e.g. renal dysfunction).

Hypertension is usually asymptomatic and picked up at a health check. Some people's BP is higher when measured by a health professional (white coat effect) due to anxiety.

Hypertension is an important contributor to several cardiovascular disorders. Several lifestyle factors are associated with hypertension, including being overweight, excess alcohol consumption, smoking and lack of exercise. Hypertension may run in families.

Diagnosis and investigations
History, examination, blood pressure monitoring (usually 24-hour ambulatory monitoring of BP instigated by the GP). Some people will record their BP at home and keep a diary.

Treatment
Hypertension is treated with lifestyle changes and/or drugs (e.g. ACE inhibitors, beta blockers, angiotensin II antagonists, calcium-channel blockers, diuretics) depending on age and ethnic origin.

Nursing care
Largely monitoring in primary care by practice nurses and advice about lifestyle modification and medication compliance.

Hysterectomy
Definition
Hysterectomy is the surgical removal of the uterus. This may or may not be accompanied by removal of the cervix and ovaries (removal of the ovaries alone is called oophorectomy).

Hysterectomy is a relatively common operation undergone by women before or after the menopause. It is usually the last resort (except when there is cancer) in a series of treatment options. Hysterectomy may be performed for the following reasons: heavy or painful periods (menorrhagia); fibroids; prolapse; endometriosis; and cancer of the uterus, cervix, fallopian tubes or ovaries.

Diagnosis and investigations
History, examination, ultrasound, biopsy.

Treatment
Varies depending on the reason for the hysterectomy. There are various types of hysterectomy:

- Total hysterectomy (removal of the uterus and cervix but not the ovaries).
- Subtotal hysterectomy (removal of the uterus).
- Radical hysterectomy (removal of the uterus, cervix, fallopian tubes, ovaries, part of the vagina and lymph nodes – usually because of cancer).

The uterus can be removed either through the vagina, through an abdominal incision or via keyhole surgery. Recovery from surgery will depend on the type of surgery performed and the reason for it. Chemotherapy or radiotherapy may follow surgery for cancer. If the ovaries are removed prior to menopause, hormone replacement therapy may be prescribed.

Nursing care
Nursing a woman having a hysterectomy should focus on the principles of pre- and post-operative care and the signs and symptoms exhibited by the person at the time. Post-operative complications may include bleeding, VTE and infection. If chemotherapy or radiotherapy is needed, nursing care will focus on these treatments and their associated side effects, as well as supporting the woman (and her family/carers) emotionally and psychologically.

Immunodeficiency
Definition
Immunodeficiency means that the immune system is deficient in some way. Immunodeficiencies can be largely classified into primary and secondary immunodeficiencies and autoimmune diseases.

People should be investigated for immunodeficiencies if they have increased susceptibility to infection. This may manifest as serious infections needing intravenous antibiotics or infections in unusual places (e.g. abscesses in the liver or brain) or infections from unusual pathogens.

There are different types of immunodeficiencies, but the most common are usually secondary to other diseases/illnesses or treatments. Primary immunodeficiency is rare (and usually diagnosed in childhood); it may result in deficiencies associated with, for example, antibodies, phagocytes, complement proteins or lymphocytes.

Autoimmune diseases occur because the immune system starts to attack the body's own cells. There are several autoimmune diseases, including Addison's disease, multiple sclerosis and rheumatoid arthritis.

Diagnosis and investigations
History, examination and relevant tests depending on presentation.

Treatment
Treatment for immunodeficiency and autoimmune diseases focuses on the underlying disease. This may include hospitalisation or be carried out in primary care.

Nursing care
The nursing care of people with immunodeficiency will depend on the severity of their disease and its underlying pathology. Nurses may have a variety of roles, ranging from health education and promotion to care of a severely immunocompromised patient in ITU. For some people treatment will focus on the presenting problem, such as poor wound healing, recurrent infections, pain or limited mobility (rheumatoid arthritis), while for others expert advice about their disease course and expectations will be needed. Nursing a person who is immunocompromised may require protective isolation.

Incontinence
Definition
Incontinence may simply be defined as passing urine or faeces in an inappropriate place. Incontinence may be transient, such as after childbirth, or it may be a continuing problem associated with odour, leakage, exposure, secrecy, embarrassment and fear of not reaching the toilet in time.

Urinary incontinence is usually categorised into different types:

- Stress urinary incontinence (SUI), which is the inability of the urethral sphincter to stay shut when pressure is exerted on the bladder by the abdomen (e.g. while sneezing, coughing or laughing, or while exercising).
- Urge incontinence, which occurs when the detrusor muscle of the bladder contracts before the person wishes it to do so.
- Mixed stress and urge incontinence.
- Overflow incontinence as a result of urinary retention (e.g. prostatic hypertrophy, faecal impaction).
- Reflex incontinence due to, for instance, spinal cord damage.
- Functional incontinence, which is when a person could be continent but cannot get to the toilet/commode in time because of, for example, mobility or cognitive problems or impaired dexterity.

Faecal incontinence may be caused by the following:

- Structural changes, including incompetent anal sphincter, pelvic floor damage (e.g. from childbirth) or haemorrhoidectomy.
- Diminished rectal sensation, for example due to diabetic neuropathy or megacolon.
- Constipation (and associated dehydration, inadequate diet, minimal exercise etc.).
- Excessive diarrhoea.
- Neurological disorders, including Parkinson's disease and multiple sclerosis.
- Cognitive impairment, such as dementia.
- Brain damage (e.g. frontal lobe carcinoma, stroke).
- Specific conditions of the bowel, including inflammatory bowel disease.

Incontinence can lead to skin excoriation and the risk of developing pressure ulcers.

Diagnosis and investigations
History, examination, routine urinalysis and referral for specialist tests, such as urodynamics.

Treatment
Depends on cause, but may include pharmacological management (e.g. in faecal incontinence making bowel evacuation more predictable by the use of bulking agents, constipating agents, suppositories or enemas); biofeedback; exercises, such as pelvic floor exercises or anal sphincter–contracting exercises; electrical stimulation of the pelvic floor; anal plugs; urethral and supra-pubic catheters, self-catheterisation, surgery or management through the use of continence aids.

Nursing care
Find out more about the person's incontinence. Take a urine specimen and test it to rule out infection. Ask about constipation and diarrhoea. Ask about any possible triggers and ways of relieving incontinence that the patient or their carers might have developed. Refer for specialist assessment. Make an assessment for pressure ulcer risk. Arrange a follow-up meeting to review the person's care and the advice/treatment given by the continence specialist.

Jaundice

Definition

Jaundice is due to raised bilirubin levels in the blood and the depositing of bile pigments in sclera, skin and mucous membranes. The signs and symptoms are skin/sclera/mucus membrane discolouration, itch, orange urine and white stools (due to intrahepatic cholestasis).

Diagnosis and investigations

History and examination. Liver function tests.

Treatment

Depends on the cause. Jaundice usually resolves in about two weeks with complete recovery.

Nursing care

Depends on the cause, but will include reassurance and hydration.

Leukaemias
Definition
Leukaemia is cancer of the blood or bone marrow. It can be acute or chronic.

Leukaemias are named after the stem-cell line that is affected, for instance in acute myeloid leukaemia (AML) the myeloid line is affected, in chronic lymphocytic leukaemia (CLL) it is the lymphoid line. The affected white blood cells (blasts) are immature and proliferate, taking over the space in the bone marrow and preventing other blood cells (e.g. red blood cells and platelets) from developing.

The main types of leukaemia affecting adults in the UK are AML and CLL. AML is associated with increasing age and peaks at around 70 years. CLL and chronic myeloid leukaemia (CML) are chronic leukaemias. The incidence of CLL increases with age, and it is more common in men. CML is rare and usually occurs in middle age.

Without treatment, acute leukaemia can progress very quickly, resulting in death within a few months. Chronic leukaemia tends to develop slowly.

Diagnosis and investigations
History, examination, blood tests and bone marrow aspiration.

Treatment
Depends on the cause, but may include blood transfusions, chemotherapy or stem-cell transplantation.

Nursing care
The nursing care of people with leukaemia will depend on its severity and the underlying pathology. For some people no treatment is needed except for advice about early signs and symptoms of infection to be alert to and to seek immediate medical advice about. Some patients undergoing chemotherapy will need care focused on relieving the side effects that they are experiencing at the time and advice about recognising the early signs of neutropenia.

Life support: advanced adult

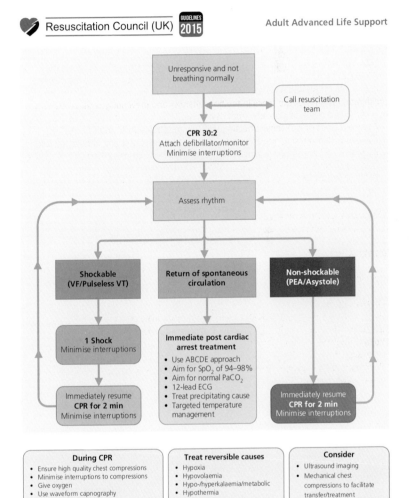

Source: Reproduced with permission of the Resuscitation Council (UK).

Life support: basic adult

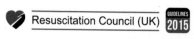 Resuscitation Council (UK) **2015**   Adult Basic Life Support

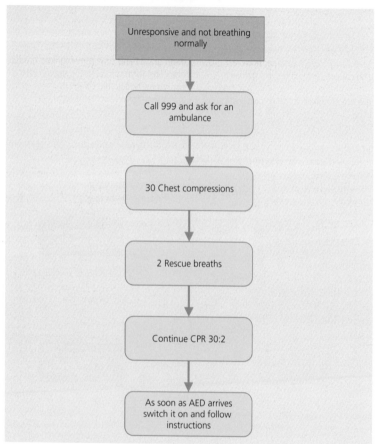

Source: Reproduced with permission of the Resuscitation Council (UK).

Lymphomas
Definition
Lymphomas are cancers of cells in the lymphatic system. There are two main types of lymphoma: Hodgkin's lymphoma and non-Hodgkin's lymphoma.

Hodgkin's lymphoma is rare, usually affecting younger adults aged between 20 and 30 years, and older people after 70 years. Hodgkin's lymphoma affects B lymphocytes. These lymphocytes collect in lymph nodes, which then get bigger and form malignant tumours. Such abnormal cells can travel to other parts of the lymphatic system, so people may develop several cancerous lymph nodes and an enlarged spleen.

Non-Hodgkin's lymphoma is a cancer affecting lymphocytes. There are several types of non-Hodgkin's lymphoma, both fast growing (high grade) and slow growing (low grade). The cancerous lymphocytes gather in lymph nodes and form tumours; they also travel within and outside the lymphatic system to other lymph nodes, the spleen and via the blood system to other parts of the body, where they form lymphoma tumours. Non-Hodgkin's lymphoma is a relatively common cancer mainly found in people over 60 years of age. Men are more commonly affected than women.

Diagnosis and investigations
Biopsy of nodes, CT and MRI scans, blood tests and bone marrow biopsy.

Treatment
Treatment will depend on type, grade and staging. Low-grade, slow-growing tumours may not require immediate treatment, but will need careful monitoring. Other, more virulent lymphomas will require treatment with chemotherapy, monoclonal antibodies or radiotherapy. Stem-cell transplants are sometimes used.

Nursing care
Nursing care is largely about delivering and monitoring responses to chemotherapy and radiotherapy, alleviating side effects of these treatments, providing psychological support, educating patients and their family/carers about drug regimens, dealing with tiredness and advising about when to seek help (e.g. infections).

Macular degeneration
Definition
Age-related macular degeneration (AMD) affects a small area of the retina called the macula, causing distortion (e.g. wavy rather than straight lines) and blurring of central vision, which may eventually progress to seeing just a blank patch. AMD will not lead to total loss of sight and is not painful, but is very distressing as it has impacts on daily living and recreational activities (e.g. reading, watching television, films, looking at photographs etc.). Regular review by an ophthalmologist is important if a person is diagnosed with AMD.

There are two types of age-related macular degeneration: wet and dry. Wet AMD is more serious but less common (~10–15% of people with AMD). In wet AMD new blood vessels replace defective ones, but they grow in the wrong place, causing bleeding and swelling below the macula and resulting in macular scarring. If untreated, wet AMD can progress quickly, causing severe damage to central vision. Rapid treatment to stop blood vessel growth is needed.

Dry AMD progresses more slowly. There is no treatment and so attention focuses on environmental changes (e.g. better lighting, magnifiers) to make the most of the remaining central vision. Referral to a low vision service linked to the local hospital/local authority may be helpful.

Diagnosis and investigations
History and examination of the eye and retina.

Treatment
Treatment for wet macular degeneration may include laser surgery to destroy the new blood vessels or injections of anti-VEGF (vascular endothelial growth factor) to prevent the growth of new blood vessels in the eye.

Nursing care
Nursing care will focus on support and referral to low vision services.

Meningitis
Definition
Meningitis is an infection of the meninges that causes the meninges to become inflamed – this may lead to damage to nerves and the brain.

Bacterial meningitis is a serious, potentially fatal infection requiring prompt diagnosis, treatment and hospitalisation. Viral meningitis is usually milder and self-limiting, however some viruses can cause severe debilitation and functional and intellectual impairment.

Some types of bacterial meningitis present with septicaemia-induced disseminated intravascular coagulation (DIC). Anyone with this type of meningitis will be seriously ill and require intensive nursing and medical care. Recovery may be prolonged and functional (e.g. because of amputations) and intellectual impairment may remain. Bacterial meningitis can have a rapid onset with symptoms including fever with cold extremities; vomiting; headache; neck stiffness; confusion and irritability; drowsiness; pale, blotchy skin, sometimes with a rash; severe muscle pain; and sensitivity to light.

Immunisation is available against some types of meningitis.

After discharge from hospital following bacterial or viral meningitis, some people continue to have minimal residual problems (e.g. headaches, poor concentration and fatigue); others may have functional deficits needing ongoing rehabilitation with physiotherapists and occupational therapists making adaptations to enable easier daily living.

Diagnosis and investigations
History, examination, lumbar puncture, blood tests.

Treatment
Depends on cause and symptoms.

Nursing care
Any infection of the CNS is debilitating and frightening. Nursing largely focuses on monitoring the patient's condition and being alert to early signs of deterioration (and progress). Management of medications and addressing symptoms are also essential.

Multiple sclerosis
Definition
Multiple sclerosis (MS) is caused by a loss of myelin in the brain and spinal cord. This compromises the passage of the nerve impulse. As myelin loss increases, more axons fail to function and permanent disabilities arise. MS is an ongoing, progressive condition that cannot be cured. It is thought to be an altered immune response to parts of the CNS. It may have genetic and/or environmental (e.g. viral or toxin) triggers. Initially, MS is generally characterised by periods of relapse and remission. This remitting/relapsing pattern is unpredictable and so can be disquieting for both the patient and their family.

As MS progresses in different ways and at different speeds in different people, it is important to care for each person as an individual and to address each of their difficulties as they occur. People with MS may experience problems such as urinary tract infections, constipation, incontinence, sexual dysfunction, muscle spasticity, mobility, unpleasant shooting pains/sensations and depression. Each will need to be addressed in a way that suits the patient and their family/carers. People with MS may also be at risk of pressure ulcers if their mobility is compromised.

Diagnosis and investigations
History, neurological examination, blood tests (to rule out other problems) and MRI scans.

Treatment
Medical treatments may focus on reducing the severity and length of acute relapses (corticosteroids may be used, although over time they may become less effective) and symptom management. Some drugs (e.g. β-interferon, copaxone) can reduce the number of relapses. Early work on monoclonal antibodies is showing positive results in relation to symptom halting.

Nursing care
Nurses in primary care and those working in the community, occupational health nurses and acute hospital nurses may all provide care to people with MS. As MS is a progressive disease, nurses providing palliative and end-of-life care may also work with people with MS and their families and carers (although MS may not significantly shorten lifespan). Nursing (and multi-disciplinary) care should focus on physical, environmental, social and psychological aspects.

Myopathies
Definition
Myopathy is a disorder of any muscle, which can lead to progressive muscle wasting and weakness. There are several types of myopathy, many of which are inherited and described as primary myopathies (e.g. Duchenne muscular dystrophy). Other myopathies may be secondary to metabolic or endocrine diseases, for instance associated with myxoedema, hyperthyroidism, Addison's disease or diabetes mellitus. Others may be linked to inflammation, such as dermatomyositis, or infection, such as HIV, or result from medications, such as statins or steroids.

Where muscle weakness is degenerative, the use of mobility aids and adaptive devices will be needed. Musculoskeletal complications from myopathies include the formation of contractures and chest and spinal deformities such as scoliosis. Occupational therapists and physiotherapists will play a major role in this element of treatment.

Diagnosis and investigations
History, examination and muscle biopsy, electromyography.

Treatment
Depends on the underlying condition.

Nursing care
Nursing care will depend on the underlying condition.

Nurses may routinely care for people with primary myopathies who need nursing care not because of their muscle weakness and related limitations, but because they are ill from another cause. In these situations care must focus on both the presenting illness and any lasting problems linked to the myopathy.

Nausea and vomiting
Definition
Nausea may be experienced on its own or be accompanied by vomiting. Nausea and vomiting are very distressing and debilitating. The key to managing these two symptoms is to work out what is causing them. This involves communication with the multi-disciplinary team, the patient and their family/carers in order to identify triggers. Nausea and vomiting may be caused by constipation, drugs, infection, dyspepsia, pain and anxiety. Vomiting might also be caused by raised intracranial pressure, tumours, blockages in the GI tract and uraemia.

Nursing care
Ask about the current episode of nausea and/or vomiting and find out if anything has triggered it (or might trigger future episodes, e.g. particular smells or foods). Avoiding triggers is important, although often difficult to achieve in a hospital ward.

Treatment for vomiting may include the patient being nil by mouth to rest the gut and relieve symptoms. If this is the case, an intravenous infusion will be sited and fluid balance monitoring will be essential. Always record vomiting and try to estimate the amount of vomit. Also note characteristics such as the presence of bile or blood, record these and report them immediately.

If the patient is not nil by mouth, make sure that something to drink is within reach and that the type of drink will not trigger further feelings of nausea or vomiting. Consider using antiemetics and discuss this with the patient and the doctor.

If nausea is associated with pain or anxiety, ensure that these symptoms are addressed.

If infection is suspected, use infection control procedures and advise the patient's family/carers about these.

Neutropenia
Definition
Neutropenia is a reduction in circulating neutrophils. Neutrophils fight infections, especially those caused by bacteria and fungi, and a low level of neutrophils puts people at risk of infection. Neutropenia can be congenital, associated with particular ethnic origins (e.g. people of African descent), acquired due to ineffective/decreased neutrophil production (e.g. in aplastic anaemia, chemotherapy, radiotherapy, alcohol abuse, HIV, bone marrow infiltration with cancer) or accelerated neutrophil turnover in blood (e.g. malaria, acute bacterial infections), an autoimmune reaction or due to thyroid dysfunction.

Mild neutropenia may result in no symptoms, but some people have mouth ulcers and oral thrush; mild/moderate neutropenia carries some risk of septicaemia; severe neutropenia is linked to septic shock and may be fatal. In mild cases treatment, with monitoring, may be carried out in primary care.

Symptoms and signs of neutropenia depend on the underlying cause and severity of the neutropenia: they may include pyrexia and obvious signs of inflammation/infection, for example around IVI line sites, or be related to specific parts of the body, such as pneumonia or rashes. These early signs of infection are important to record and report. For instance, a temperature of 37.5 °C or more in cancer-linked neutropenia may be the first sign of a person developing febrile neutropenia, which can rapidly progress to sepsis.

The Multinational Association for Supportive Care in Cancer (MASCC) has produced a risk assessment tool for use with people with cancer who are at risk of developing febrile neutropenia.

In people with febrile neutropenia, early treatment (within 30 minutes of being alerted) is critical to their survival – neutropenic sepsis is a medical emergency. Rapid treatment of the underlying cause and prevention of shock are key, and this necessitates hospitalisation.

Nursing care
The nursing care of people with neutropenia will depend on its severity and the underlying pathology. For some people no treatment will be required except for advice about early signs and symptoms of infection to be alert to and to seek immediate medical advice about. Some patients undergoing chemotherapy that might induce neutropenia are advised to seek early advice if their temperature is raised, they feel unwell, or they have a sore throat, pain urinating, coughs/breathlessness or redness/swelling around an infusion site.

Osteoarthritis

Definition

Osteoarthritis is a progressive degenerative joint disease. It is the most common joint disease found in older people. Osteoarthritis is characterised by progressive cartilage damage and loss together with changes in the nearby bones due to the formation of osteophytes (bony projections/spurs).

Signs and symptoms include joint pain (insidious onset with usually slow progression to severe) aggravated by activity and relieved by rest, joint stiffness ('gelling' after inactivity) and bony swellings, especially in the hands, all of which lead to a reduced range of movement in the affected joints.

Diagnosis and investigations

History and examination.

Treatment

Treatment centres on maintaining function and symptom management. This will include pain relief tailored to the individual's needs (which may include injections of corticosteroids into joints), physiotherapy and occupational therapy focusing on exercises and adaptations for daily living. Weight loss may be advised and surgical replacement of joints (e.g. knee, hip) may be considered.

Nursing care

Nursing care will depend on the severity, location and treatment of the osteoarthritis, but will likely focus on pain management, advice about weight loss and healthy eating if necessary, and mobility. Pre- and post-operative care will be needed if joint replacement surgery is undertaken. It is important that nurses work closely with the patient and with the multi-disciplinary team.

Osteomyelitis
Definition
Osteomyelitis is an infection of the bone. It may result from an open (compound) fracture or spread via the circulatory system. Osteomyelitis is rare in adults; when it occurs it may be linked to an infection with staphylococcus, infections related to diabetes and diabetic foot infections, spinal TB (tuberculosis) or hospital-acquired septicaemia from IVI lines.

Diagnosis and investigations
History, examination and blood tests.

Treatment
Treatment centres on treating the infection.

Nursing care
Nursing care will depend on the severity, location and treatment of the infection.

Osteoporosis
Definition
Osteoporosis is a condition in which bones lose their density and become weak and brittle, meaning that they are more likely to break easily. It is found most commonly in older women, but also occurs in men.

In women, osteoporosis is associated with oestrogen withdrawal, for instance following menopause – especially if early menopause, late menarche or if women have had a long history of oligomenorrhoea (athletes, women who have/had anorexia nervosa). Other risk factors include smoking, excessive alcohol consumption, steroid use, a sedentary lifestyle or a family history of osteoporosis.

Osteoporosis can also be a result of another disease, including thyrotoxicosis, Cushing's disease or cirrhosis of the liver.

Diagnosis and investigations
History, examination, bone density measurement.

Treatment
Treatment for osteoporosis will include lifestyle advice and supplements of calcium and vitamin D. Hormonal therapy may be considered.

Nursing care
Nursing care will largely focus on health education and health promotion, and if necessary care related to fractures. Practice nurses and other public health nurses should emphasise the importance of preventing osteoporosis through continued health education and promotion of good bone health – this will include advice about taking regular weight-bearing exercise (e.g. brisk walking, dancing, aerobics, tennis), eating a balanced, varied diet and ensuring adequate vitamin D levels (vitamin D helps to absorb calcium). Being outside in the sun is the best way to get vitamin D, but if this is not possible vitamin D supplements may be taken. Advice may also relate to smoking cessation and minimising the risk of tripping or falling (being aware of hazards both in and out of the home and also underlying health problems that might cause dizziness).

Pain and discomfort

Definition

Pain and discomfort are distressing and debilitating symptoms; both are very individual experiences and need to be treated as such. Pain has physical, emotional and sociocultural components and can be influenced by the environment in which it is experienced and also the other people involved in that experience (e.g. family, carers, nurses).

Pain can be acute or chronic (or on a continuum between the two), and may be experienced on its own or be accompanied by other symptoms that will also need to be alleviated.

Acute pain usually has a limited onset and points to a clear cause.

Chronic pain is prolonged, lasting beyond the course of an acute disease or healing associated with it. Chronic pain can have impacts on a person's life in many ways, for instance causing isolation, debilitation, altered lifestyle, altered personality, depression and reduced functional ability.

Managing pain, as with other symptoms, involves working out what is causing it and how best to alleviate it. This requires communication with the patient and their family/carers and the multi-disciplinary team.

Nursing care

Effective assessment and management of pain are key components of nursing care. Pain must be assessed thoroughly and regularly if it is to be managed well. Pain may be assessed using pain scales (e.g. pain rulers, visual analogue scales, 'smiley faces', body maps), but talking about pain is just as important. Anxiety exacerbates pain, so careful explanation of procedures and the cause of pain are important.

Different types of pain require different approaches to their management. For instance, surgical pain can be anticipated and a plan to manage it should be made prior to surgery whenever possible. In pre-existing pain it is important to find out more about the current episode of pain (e.g. location, intensity), what triggered it, how the patient usually manages and copes with it and what they have tried to alleviate the pain with what effect.

In chronic pain it is useful to consider other factors that might have an impact on the pain and contribute to a lowered pain threshold, and those that might be affected by the pain (e.g. anxiety, depression, lifestyle, functional ability, fatigue, family/carers' reactions and tolerance).

Pain assessment in vulnerable groups of people needs to be handled sensitively and innovatively (e.g. older people with dementia, people whose attitude to pain may be to put up with it, people with learning disabilities who may find it hard to express themselves, people who are confused or unconscious). Appropriate communication is a central feature of effective pain management.

There are various approaches that can be used to achieve successful pain management, pharmacological (analgesics) or non-pharmacological. Non-pharmacological management includes information giving, relaxation techniques, meditation, hypnosis, acupuncture, TENS (transcutaneous electrical nerve stimulation), heat/cold therapies and therapies that result in distraction, such as those involving art, music or guided imagery. Non-pharmacological and pharmacological techniques can be combined.

Pancreatitis
Definition
Pancreatitis is inflammation of the pancreas. It is associated with auto-digestion of pancreatic tissue, leading to oedema, bleeding and necrosis. Signs and symptoms depend on the severity of the inflammation. In mild or moderate pancreatitis there is constant upper abdominal pain of sudden onset; the pain may radiate through to the back; nausea and maybe vomiting, pyrexia and jaundice may be present. In severe pancreatitis pain will be severe, and hypovolaemic shock and compromised respiration and kidney function may occur.

Pancreatitis can be acute or chronic. Most pancreatitis resolves spontaneously, although severe pancreatitis can be life threatening.

Acute pancreatitis is most commonly caused by gallstones, or over-consumption of alcohol. Rarer causes include trauma, drugs (e.g. oestrogen, corticosteroids), viral infection (e.g. mumps, coxsackie) and hyperlipidaemia. Sometimes there is no known cause (idiopathic). Complications of acute pancreatitis include abscesses, intra-abdominal sepsis, necrosis of the transverse colon, respiratory (type 1) and renal failure, pancreatic haemorrhage and cardiac arrhythmias if electrolyte balance is disturbed. Secondary diabetes mellitus may occur.

Chronic pancreatitis is usually caused by alcohol abuse leaving residual damage to the pancreas following acute pancreatitis. Exocrine and endocrine pancreatic insufficiency (causing diabetes and steatorrhoea) is associated with chronic pancreatitis.

Diagnosis and investigations
Examination, history, blood tests (amylase levels usually raised), ultrasound or CT scan.

Treatment
Mild/moderate pancreatitis is usually managed by IV fluids, nil by mouth, analgesia and recording of vital signs for early detection of deterioration. Severe pancreatitis usually requires care in HDU/ITU with invasive monitoring. Surgery is only used to treat severe complications. In some instances pancreatic enzyme supplementation is needed.

Nursing care
Nursing care will depend on the severity of the pancreatitis, but will always need to focus on symptom control and management, as well as accurate assessment and regular monitoring. Pain, anxiety, nausea and vomiting are likely to be the patient's main problems. Nurses should particularly monitor the patient for signs of hypovolaemic shock (due to excessive vomiting, bleeding), arrhythmias, respiratory failure and alterations to blood glucose levels. Help with daily living activities will be needed for patients who are acutely ill.

If a patient has chronic pancreatitis, most of their care will be provided in primary care. In this situation practice nurses will largely be responsible for providing advice about pain relief and lifestyle changes (e.g. avoiding alcohol consumption, smoking cessation, changing to a low-fat diet). Diabetes may be a complication of chronic pancreatitis, so advice should be given about recognising symptoms of diabetes and its management.

Parkinson's disease

Definition

Parkinson's disease (PD) is caused by a loss in the brain of dopamine-producing cells in the substantia nigra and the presence of Lewy bodies. Lewy bodies are small proteins that alter the action of dopamine and acetylcholine. Dopamine is essential for the control of movement, posture and coordination. PD is characterised by slow movements, resting tremor, rigidity and postural instability. All of these may result in falls. For some people intellectual deterioration, incontinence and constipation can also occur.

PD is usually associated with increased age. Some types of PD may be linked to particular gene mutations and some types are hereditary.

PD will progress differently in different people, so it is important to care for each person as an individual and to address each of their difficulties as it occurs.

PD-like symptoms may also be a side effect of some drugs, including antiemetics, neuroleptics and lithium. Stopping the drug should stop the symptoms.

Diagnosis and investigations

Examination, history (falls may be the reason for consultation) and brain imaging.

Treatment

PD cannot be cured and is a progressive disease. Symptoms can usually be controlled by treatments that increase dopamine levels in the CNS. L-dopa may be one treatment; others may focus on stimulating CNS dopamine receptors (e.g. dopamine agonists).

Drug side effects such as involuntary movement disorders (dyskinesia) can occur. In some people dopamine agonists may induce bizarre side effects, such as excessive gambling and hypersexuality, and so their impact should be monitored carefully.

Nursing care

Nursing (and multi-disciplinary) care should focus on physical, environmental, social and psychological aspects of care relevant to each individual. Nurses in primary care and those working in the community, occupational health nurses and acute hospital nurses may all provide care to people with PD. As PD is a progressive disease, nurses providing palliative and end-of-life care may also become involved.

Peptic ulceration
Definition
Peptic ulceration can occur in either the stomach (gastric ulcer) or the duodenum (duodenal ulcer). Ulcers form when gastric acid production exceeds normal amounts and causes mucosal damage. Helicobacter pylori damage the mucosal defence system and are therefore associated with ulceration.

Risk factors include the use of gastric irritants such as aspirin and NSAIDs. Smoking is also linked to ulcer development. Symptoms associated with peptic ulceration are pain (dyspepsia) and sometimes vomiting; often a patient has no symptoms prior to a gastro-intestinal haemorrhage. A gastro-intestinal haemorrhage is a medical emergency.

Complications of peptic ulceration include vomiting, bleeding (haematemesis/malaena), perforation and peritonitis. Some gastric ulcers may be early gastric cancer, so biopsy is important.

Diagnosis and investigations
History, examination, blood and breath tests and endoscopy.

Treatment
Treatment includes combinations of drugs to reduce gastric acid, eradicate helicobacter pylori and, if unsatisfactory or the ulcer has perforated, surgery.

Nursing care
Nursing people with peptic ulceration can span community and hospital care. Management with medication prescribed by the GP may be the first course of treatment for patients with peptic ulceration.

Gastro-intestinal haemorrhage is an emergency and will require prompt nursing care if a patient is in hospital or if at home, prompt advice to call for an emergency ambulance. If a patient requires surgery, the principles of pre- and post-operative care should be adhered to.

Surgery is likely to be done as an emergency and the patient (and their family/carers) will be feeling vulnerable and afraid. Caring for them will require highly skilled communication as well as attentive, accurate assessment and monitoring.

Peripheral vascular disease
Definition
Peripheral vascular disease includes arterial and venous disease. Arterial and venous disease can occur separately or together.

Peripheral arterial disease (PAD) is commonly caused by arteriosclerosis. In PAD, reduction in blood flow to peripheral tissues results in acute or chronic ischaemia. PAD affects 10% of the population over 65 years of age in the western world.

Peripheral venous disease (PVD) occurs because of obstruction (e.g. thrombus or thrombophlebitis) or venous valve incompetence.

Risk factors for peripheral vascular disease include smoking, hypertension, hyperlipidaemia, diabetes mellitus and family history.

Signs and symptoms of chronic PAD include claudication (aching pain in leg after walking, relieved by rest), cold peripheries, prolonged capillary refill time, rest pain at night, absent pulses depending on location of diseased artery, arterial ulcers (over pressure points – heels, toes) and erectile dysfunction. In acute PAD pain can be sudden and severe, skin is pale/mottled and the limb is cold. Pins and needles or paralysis can be present and pulses are altered, being weak or absent.

Signs and symptoms of chronic PVD include foot to calf oedema, warm peripheries, and legs that are brownish/red in colour, possibly cyanosed and often mottled. Varicose veins may be visible and there may be ulcers at the ankles. Legs may feel heavy and full. In acute PVD there is minimal pain, but there may be tenderness along the course of an inflamed vein.

Leg ulcers are associated with both PAD and PVD.

Complications may be associated with coronary heart disease for those with PAD and pulmonary embolism and deep vein thrombosis for those with PVD.

Diagnosis and investigations
History, examination and ultrasound assessments.

Treatment
Depends on presenting problems and diagnosis.

Nursing care
Nursing care will largely focus on both lifestyle advice and medication monitoring for those with non-disabling PAD, or pre- and post-operative care for those requiring surgery (e.g. balloon angioplasty and stent insertion, bypass surgery, surgical embolectomy or amputation). In PVD nursing care, from practice nurses or community nurses, will largely focus on assessing and monitoring progress and ulcer management. Some ulcers will not heal and will require grafting in hospital.

Platelet disorders

Definition

Platelets are very small blood cells (thrombocytes) produced in the bone marrow. They have no nucleus and live for around 5–9 days. Dead platelets are removed by macrophages in the spleen and liver. A platelet's surface contains proteins that allow it to adhere to other proteins (e.g. collagen). Platelets are important in clotting and preventing blood loss – they are therefore central to maintaining haemostasis.

Disorders of platelets are linked to excessive bleeding (low numbers) or thrombosis (high numbers), resulting in VTE, strokes and myocardial infarctions.

Thrombocytopenia is a reduction in the number of platelets. This may be because too few platelets are produced or too many platelets are destroyed. Underproduction is usually linked to aplastic anaemia or bone marrow damage due to, for instance, leukaemia, lymphoma, vitamin B12 or folate deficiency, or HIV infection. Excess destruction can be linked to viral or bacterial infection, liver disease, disseminated intravascular coagulation (DIC), connective tissue disease (e.g. systemic lupus erythematosus) or hypersplenism. Thrombocytopenia presents as purpura, petechiae, mucosal bleeding, nose bleeds or heavy periods.

Thrombocytosis is an increase in platelets. This can occur in myeloproliferative disease, for example essential thrombocythaemia, or be secondary to anaemia or inflammation. The risk associated with thrombocytosis largely lies in the risk of thrombosis development. Prophylaxis against thrombosis (e.g. aspirin) should be given, as well as advice about identifying signs and symptoms of a deep vein thrombosis (DVT)/pulmonary embolus (PE).

Diagnosis and investigations

History, examination and blood tests.

Treatment

Treatment depends on the underlying pathology.

Nursing care

The nursing care of people with platelet disorders will depend on the type and severity of the disease. For some people no treatment will be required, except for advice about things to avoid (e.g. contact sports, aspirin preparations, needle-stick injury or cuts) and carrying clear medic alerts to draw attention to their illness. Others will require prophylaxis with aspirin if they have a risk of thrombosis. Some patients may be very ill (e.g. with DIC or liver disease) and require specialist hospitalised care.

Pneumonia
Definition
Pneumonia is an acute, infective respiratory illness of the lungs that is caused by viruses, bacteria or fungi. There are four main types: community-acquired pneumonia, hospital-acquired (nosocomial) pneumonia, aspiration pneumonia and pneumonia in immunocompromised people.

Fever, cough, chest pain and breathlessness are common symptoms. Some people also have headaches, confusion, myalgia and malaise.

Most people with community-acquired pneumonia are cared for at home, but some will require hospitalisation if their symptoms deteriorate.

Vaccination is available against pneumonia and is advised for all people over 65 years of age or those with long-term respiratory conditions.

Diagnosis and investigations
History, examination, pulse oximetry and blood tests.

Treatment
Treatment may include antibiotics, oxygen therapy, intravenous fluid therapy and nutritional support. Physiotherapy may also be necessary.

Nursing care
The nursing care of patients with pneumonia, whether in primary care or in hospital, needs to be observant and vigilant. Care focuses on monitoring temperature, pulse, respirations and blood pressure, administering oxygen as prescribed, helping with activities of daily living, ensuring adequate fluid intake and nutrition, relieving breathlessness through positioning (leaning forward in bed on a bed table supported by pillows or just sitting forward in a chair), and helping the person to expectorate sputum with or without the assistance of the physiotherapist. A patient's condition can deteriorate rapidly and if it happens, this needs swift medical attention.

Post-operative care
Definition
Post-operative care commences once the patient is returned to the ward routine after an operation. It includes regular observations of vital signs (pulse, blood pressure, temperature and respirations), checking the wound/drains for bleeding (dressings soaked with blood indicate excessive bleeding), checking for ischaemia, recording fluid intake and output, ensuring that pain is managed appropriately, noting and reporting any unusual behaviours (confusion, restlessness), ensuring that nausea and/or vomiting are managed appropriately, coaxing the patient to drink and noting their tolerance of fluids, and encouraging the patient to pass urine if no catheter is inserted or following its removal. Deviations from the norm should be reported immediately. For example, decreased blood pressure may suggest hypovolaemic shock (e.g. due to bleeding or vomiting), increased pulse may suggest low circulating blood levels (e.g. due to bleeding). (N.B. Increased respiratory rate coupled with shallow breathing may occur before tachycardia and hypotension are noted.)

If gastro-intestinal surgery has been performed, peristalsis usually returns to normal after about 48 hours and meals/snacks should only be introduced after confirmation with the medical team. Patients may describe cramps, wind or hunger as bowel function returns. Listening for bowel sounds with a stethoscope may be required following GI tract surgery.

Once the immediate post-operative period is over and the patient is feeling hungry, easily digestible food (and fluid) should be gradually re-introduced. Monitoring the patient's tolerance of food is important. Small, frequent meals may be better tolerated than large meals. Establishing good nutrition is essential for healing.

Wound care is an important facet of post-operative care, as is ensuring strict infection control procedures.

Encouraging mobility and deep breathing exercises are essential in reducing the likelihood of VTE. However, a person in pain is unlikely to want to move, so mobilisation and pain management should be considered alongside each other.

Remember to discuss the patient's progress with them and their family/carers. An encouraging and realistic approach is important during the recovery period and can help alleviate anxiety, encourage compliance with post-operative instructions and exercises and build the patient's (and the family's) confidence in preparation for discharge from the ward.

Specific post-operative care may be necessary for certain operations. You should check if this is the case with senior colleagues, doctors and specialist nurses to ensure that the right specialist preparation or care is carried out.

Pre- and intra-operative care
Definition
Avoiding harm and keeping people safe before, during and after surgery are critical components of nursing. Pre-operative care is the physical and psychological care provided to a patient (and their family/carers) prior to surgery. Intra-operative care is provided during surgery by theatre nurses, operating department technicians, anaesthetists and surgeons. Post-operative care (see previous section) is care provided following surgery in the theatre recovery area and on the ward.

Pre-operatively, assessments need to be made of the patient's physical condition and their risk of developing venous thromboembolism (anti-embolic stockings applied appropriately and prophylaxis given as prescribed), pressure ulcers (pressure-relieving equipment available), pulmonary aspiration (due to inhaling gastric contents during the induction of anaesthesia or during surgical manipulations; fasting procedure instituted correctly), surgical site infections or difficulties closing skin/applying dressings (removal of hair as appropriate using clippers or depilation creams rather than shaving, which risks cutting the skin), toxic shock syndrome in women who are menstruating and using tampons (discuss using sanitary pads rather than tampons during surgery; if tampons are left in situ for more than 6 hours infection may develop), or allergic reactions to products used during surgery (e.g. latex gloves, skin cleansing fluids, dressings, dressing tapes).

Attention should also be paid pre-operatively to increasing the patient's knowledge about the surgery and its consequences and alleviating anxiety by listening to concerns and giving simple and truthful information. Family and carers will also be anxious. Check that consent has been given for surgery (usually obtained by the surgeon); that the patient is wearing an identification band with their name and hospital number clearly marked; that an allergy band is worn if appropriate; that the operation site has been clearly marked by the surgeon; and that the right patient is taken for surgery together with all of their relevant documentation.

Intra-operative care starts once the patient has been handed over to the theatre staff and continues until the patient is discharged from the recovery suite. Specific checks are made in the anaesthetic room and the operating theatre to safeguard the patient prior to surgery. Primarily these relate to ensuring that the right patient is being operated on, the right operation is about to be performed, any risks associated with the operation have been recognised (e.g. amount of blood loss) and any risks associated with the patient (e.g. previous medical history, allergies, risk of VTE) have been recognised. After the operation is completed and before the patient leaves the operating theatre, more checks are made. These focus on the equipment used, any tests/specimens taken, the information recorded about the procedure, any problems experienced and instructions to be carried out during the immediate post-operative recovery period. Following surgery, patients are cared for in the recovery suite attached to the theatre until their condition is stable and they are conscious.

Specific pre-operative care may be necessary for certain operations. You should check if this is the case with senior colleagues, doctors and specialist nurses to ensure that the right specialist preparation or care is carried out.

Prostate gland disorders

Definition

Prostate disorders are a common problem for men over the age of 60 years. They largely fall into two groups: benign prostatic hypertrophy and prostatic cancer. Benign prostatic hypertrophy often presents with problems associated with urination (e.g. hesitancy, dribbling, frequency, incontinence or more acutely retention of urine). Prostate cancer is common in older men and is often slow growing. Prostate cancer may also present with bladder problems.

Diagnosis and investigations

History, examination and blood tests.

Treatment

Surgery may be a treatment option for both benign prostatic hypertrophy and prostate cancer.

In cancer, either a resection of the prostate (transurethral resection of the prostate, TURP) or prostatectomy may be performed, depending on the disease's progression. While TURP may improve symptoms, quality of life and life expectancy for men with cancer, it can also cause retrograde ejaculation (semen is ejaculated into the bladder), resulting in a dry orgasm. There is also a low risk of impotence and temporary incontinence. All of these risks should be discussed with the person (and their partner) beforehand. Prostatectomy has a larger risk of impotence.

Nursing care

Apart from the obvious fear of cancer, prostatic disorders can be distressing because of their interference with usual activities of daily living. Nurses need to be sensitive to this and to the possibility of embarrassment around the discussion of urinary and sexual difficulties; communication should be straightforward and informative. Some people will require advice about continence. Catheter care is important if a catheter has been inserted following acute retention of urine to avoid introducing infection.

If a patient requires surgery, nursing care will focus on the principles of pre- and post-operative care. Post-operative complications may include bleeding (haematuria), clot retention in the bladder and urethra, VTE and infection.

Psoriasis
Definition
Psoriasis presents with inflamed, reddened, silver-scaled lesions, usually on extensor surfaces of the body (e.g. knees, elbows). Psoriasis can be mild or severe and is exacerbated by stress, infections, smoking, some medications (e.g. anti-malarials), sunlight, hormonal changes (puberty and menopause) and alcohol. There are several types.

Guttate psoriasis is linked to a sore throat and small patches of psoriasis occur over the body. It can last from a few weeks to a few months, then often disappears.

Generalised pustular and erythrodermic psoriasis can be a very serious condition resulting in skin failure and requiring hospitalisation. Skin failure can lead to failure of thermoregulation, fluid loss and infection.

Some people with psoriasis may have psoriatic arthritis, which results in painful and swollen joints.

Diagnosis
History and examination.

Treatment
Treatment for psoriasis includes keeping the skin moisturised, vitamin D–based treatments and corticosteroids.

Some people with severe psoriasis may be treated with phototherapy with UVB (ultraviolet B) light.

Nursing care
Nursing care will depend on the severity of psoriasis and may range from advice about medications to more intensive care related to skin failure. If skin failure has occurred then care should focus on the close monitoring of thermoregulation (warmth, management of pyrexia and rigours), loss of fluid through the skin (oral fluids), fluid balance (input and output), nutritional intake (loss of protein – refer to dietician), pain (analgesics), deterioration (e.g. infection; level of consciousness; cardiac function – heart rate, respiratory rate, BP).

Any deterioration of skin or other systems should be reported immediately.

Raised intracranial pressure
Definition
Raised intracranial pressure is a medical emergency. Head injuries or other pathologies, either intracranial (e.g. cerebral abscess, haematomas or other space-occupying lesions such as malignant or benign tumours) or extracranial (e.g. hepatic encephalopathy), may cause the pressure in the skull to rise, which in turn may result in coma, irreversible brain damage or death.

Nursing care
Common signs and symptoms of raised intracranial pressure of which nurses need to be aware and act on immediately are:

- Any alterations in consciousness.
- Focal neurological deficits, e.g. limb weakness or speech deficits, pupil changes, double vision.

Alterations to vital signs such as slowed and irregular respiratory rate, slowed heart rate and increased blood pressure may follow, but are not always the first signs to be present. An elevated temperature may occur due to compression of the hypothalamus. Check observations and record your assessment against the Early Warning System/Glasgow Coma Scale. Call for immediate help, stay with the patient and monitor closely.

Ongoing nursing care will depend largely on medical treatment and the patient's condition, but may include the following:

- Accurate, frequent monitoring of vital signs (+ intracranial pressure, if measured, – normal limits equal to or less than 15 mmHg). Be alert to changes in respiration, blood pressure and pulse. Changes to the cardiovascular system will mean less blood reaching the already compromised brain. Report alterations in BP (systolic < 90 or > 160 mmHg; diastolic < 50 or > 100 mmHg) and pulse (<50 or > 100 beats/minute).
- Maintenance of the airway.
- Accurate assessment and monitoring of level of consciousness; be alert to even the slightest change (e.g. agitation, restlessness, taking longer to respond than before).
- Care of infusions and urinary catheter and infection control.
- Administration of prescribed medications.
- Skilled, reassuring communication with the patient and their family/carers regardless of the patient's level of consciousness.
- Rapid communication of deterioration to the medical team.
- If surgery is needed, post-operative observations should focus on continuous assessment of neurological state and immediate reporting of alterations, as well as giving appropriate medications.

Respiratory failure
Definition
Respiratory failure means that the body's cells do not receive adequate amounts of oxygen for survival and/or cannot offload enough CO_2 (carbon dioxide). Respiratory failure is defined by abnormal levels of arterial oxygen (low) or carbon dioxide (high). There are two types of respiratory failure: type I (hypoxaemia) and type II (hypercapnia with hypoxaemia).

Hypoxaemia refers to lack of oxygen in arterial blood due to a failure of oxygenation ($PaO_2 < 8kPa$).

Hypercapnia refers to excess carbon dioxide in arterial blood due to a failure of respiration ($PaCO_2 > 6kPa$).

Respiratory failure can be acute, chronic or acute on chronic.

Respiratory failure can result from, for instance, underlying lung pathology, respiratory muscle weakness or exhaustion or depressed breathing, as in drug overdose.

Excess CO_2 reduces O_2 binding to haemoglobin in the lungs, increasing the chance of hypoxaemia. Excess CO_2 in type II respiratory failure can disturb the acid-base balance. (N.B. If arterial blood pH deviates from its normal range of 7.35–7.45, an acid-base imbalance results, which is known as an acidosis [<7.35] or alkalosis [>7.45].)

Respiratory acidosis occurs when excessive arterial CO_2 in type II respiratory failure causes arterial blood pH to fall below 7.35.

Potential respiratory failure can sometimes be averted, so nurses should be alert for early warning signs of respiratory failure (restlessness, confusion, increased rate of breathing with greater effort and use of respiratory and abdominal muscles, changed patterns of breathing, flaring of the nostrils and pale or cyanosed, clammy skin) and call for medical advice immediately. If left untreated the patient's condition will deteriorate, resulting in coma and death.

Patients with respiratory failure should be monitored in a high-dependency area (respiratory rate, ECG, pulse oximetry, BP, arterial blood gas analysis, Glasgow Coma Scale).

Diagnosis and investigations
Diagnosis is made by the measurement of arterial blood gases (measuring pH is also important).

Treatment
Depending on the cause, treatment may include oxygen therapy, continuous positive airway pressure (CPAP) or intubation and mechanical ventilation.

Nursing care
Nursing care involves careful monitoring of the patient's condition and ensuring that treatment is given as prescribed. Any deterioration of the patient's condition should be reported immediately.

Care should be taken when nursing patients with COPD and chronic hypoxia, since they rely on reduced O_2 rather than higher CO_2 to drive respiration (hypoxic drive); giving oxygen may remove the drive and stop them breathing.

Rheumatoid arthritis
Definition
Rheumatoid arthritis (RA) is a systemic autoimmune disorder. The effects range from mild to severe (e.g. joint swelling, pain, stiffness and tenderness). The smaller joints of the hands, feet and wrists tend to be affected first, with subsequent involvement of larger joints. Tenosynovitis may be present.

Although RA commonly centres on joints, extra-articular signs may be present, including splinter haemorrhages in nails and skin ulceration due to vasculitis; there may also be kidney, lung and heart involvement.

Rheumatoid arthritis is more common in younger women than younger men, but by 65 years of age there is no difference between the sexes.

Diagnosis
History, examination, joint imaging and blood tests, including for erythrocyte sedimentation rate (ESR) and C-reactive protein (CRP), and rheumatoid factor and anti-CCP antibodies.

Treatment
Treatment will include tailored rehabilitation and pain relief to minimise symptoms and improve prognosis. This requires multi-disciplinary involvement (physiotherapy for e.g. exercise and local symptomatic treatment; occupational therapy for e.g. splinting and aids/adaptations). Treatment will also focus on achieving disease remission, for instance through treatment with disease-modifying antirheumatic drugs (DMARDs); corticosteroids may be given to control symptoms until DMARDs work. Surgical joint stabilisation or replacement may be needed.

Nursing care
Nursing care will depend on the severity of the disease and the treatment prescribed. It is likely to include discussions of pain management, activities of daily living and the usefulness of modifications, and pre- and post-operative care if joint replacement surgery is required. Working closely with the multi-disciplinary team will always be essential.

Sepsis
Definition
Sepsis is an infection with a systemic response – raised or lowered temperature (>38 °C or < 36 °C), increased respiratory rate (>20 breaths/minute), tachycardia (>90 beats/minute) and a raised or lowered white blood cell count. Recognising and responding to these signs are vital in preventing a rapid deterioration in a patient's condition, with the possibility of progression to septic shock.

Sepsis can occur for many reasons (e.g. bacterial or fungal infections, poor resistance/increased susceptibility to infection, a response to surgery or a wound infection, a result of infection from invasive procedures such as IV infusions or urinary catheters).

Septic shock is sepsis with organ dysfunction and hypotension despite adequate fluid resuscitation. It may manifest in acute confusional state, coma, adult respiratory distress syndrome (ARDS), circulatory failure, acute renal failure or haemostatic failure.

Diagnosis
History, examination and relevant blood (and other) tests.

Treatment
Care focuses on treating the cause and presenting signs and symptoms and evaluating organ function for deterioration (or improvement).

Nursing care
Nursing care will be in direct response to medical intervention (e.g. administration of antibiotics, management of IVIs) and monitoring vital signs. Accurate, frequent monitoring and reporting of vital signs are critical.

Shock

Definition

Shock is a medical emergency that shows itself by hypoperfusion and reduced tissue oxygenation. Reduced tissue oxygenation causes aerobic metabolism to change to anaerobic, resulting in lactic acidosis or metabolic acidosis (serum pH decreased).

Shock is associated with multi-system failure and high mortality.

There are several different types of shock: cardiogenic, obstructive, distributive and hypovolaemic. All have consequences for the cardiovascular system.

People at risk of shock include those with chest pain (or post-MI), cardiac arrhythmias, infections (including those acquired in hospital), multiple trauma, severe burns, haemorrhage (e.g. GI tract, post-operative or post-partum) and multiple allergies.

Diagnosis and investigations

History, examination and relevant blood (and other) tests.

Common signs and symptoms of shock of which nurses need to be aware and act on immediately are:

- Low systolic BP < 90 mmHg.
- Alterations to heart rate (e.g. rapid, weak, thready pulse in cardiogenic shock; bounding pulse in distributive shock).
- Increased respiratory rate.
- Cool (sweaty) skin.
- Cyanosis.
- Dizziness, agitation, lethargy.
- Confusion.
- Low urine output.
- Obvious loss of blood (e.g. post-operative, GI tract bleed).
- Excessive diarrhoea or vomiting.
- Pain.
- Abnormal blood gases and electrolytes.
- Unresponsive hypoglycaemia.

Treatment

Management varies depending on the type of shock, but the aim of treatment is always to maximise the perfusion of vital organs. Treatment focuses on treating the cause and presenting signs and symptoms and evaluating organ function for deterioration (or improvement).

Nursing care

Nurses need to be alert to the early signs and symptoms of shock. In cases where shock might be likely, regular assessment against an Early Warning System is imperative so that immediate help can be summoned. Always stay with the patient and monitor them closely. Ongoing nursing care will depend largely on medical treatment and the patient's condition, but will include accurate, frequent monitoring of vital signs (+ ECG) and oxygen saturation, fluid intake and output, level of consciousness and pain. Care of infusions and urinary catheter and infection control are also important, as is the appropriate administration of prescribed medications and oxygen. Skilled, reassuring communication with the patient and their family/carers is vital. Any deterioration/alteration needs to be communicated rapidly to the medical team.

Spinal cord compression
Definition
Acute spinal cord compression is a medical emergency. Spinal cord compression may occur because of, for example, secondary tumours from breast, prostate or lung cancers; prolapsed intervertebral discs or abscesses; or other inflammatory lesions.

Acute spinal cord compression presents with rapidly deteriorating motor dysfunction, largely of the lower limbs. If this happens to any of your patients, call for immediate medical assistance or an emergency ambulance.

Diagnosis and investigations
Diagnosis is usually made by MRI scanning.

Treatment
Depends on cause – if possible, surgical decompression.

Nursing care
Initial nursing care is likely to focus on rapid preparation for surgery. Remain calm and give clear explanations and information to the patient and their family/carers. Ongoing care will involve specialised post-operative care and support that will depend on the nature of any residual problems.

Tension pneumothorax
Definition
Tension pneumothorax is a medical emergency. A pneumothorax is when air leaks into the pleural space. There are various types of pneumothorax, but the most rapidly life threatening is a tension pneumothorax. In this instance the leak creates a one-way valve, drawing air into the pleural space that cannot escape. The increased volume of air in the pleural space causes an increase in pressure above atmospheric pressure, resulting in compression of the lung and movement of the mediastinum and heart towards the opposite side (a mediastinal shift). This reduces cardiac filling and output.

Tension pneumothorax results in severe dyspnoea, tracheal deviation (movement), tachycardia and hypotension. If unrecognised and untreated, death will occur.

A tension pneumothorax may result from trauma, asthma or chronic lung disease such as COPD.

Diagnosis
History and examination.

Treatment
Treatment is by aspiration and the insertion of a chest tube and an underwater-sealed chest drain. (The underwater-sealed drain acts as a one-way valve, allowing air to escape from the pleural cavity during expiration but not to be drawn back, since the end of the tube is covered with water.)

Nursing care
Reassurance and explanation will be important. Ensure that drains are kept below the level of the patient's chest so that water does not enter the pleural cavity.

Tinnitus
Definition
Tinnitus refers to hearing sounds that come from inside the body and is often described as ringing in the ears. It can be transient or permanent. Although tinnitus is rarely a sign of a serious underlying condition, for some people it causes considerable distress, insomnia and sometimes depression. Tinnitus usually subsides with time, but may be associated with ear infections or an accumulation of ear wax, and so checking it out is important.

Diagnosis
History and examination.

Treatment
Depends on the cause. Referral to an audiologist/ENT (ear, nose and throat) specialist may be needed and treatment may include sound therapy (listening to neutral sounds to distract from the sound of tinnitus), psychological therapies and counselling to help people to cope with tinnitus and make it less noticeable.

Nursing care
Reassurance and explanation will be important. Advice about wax removal may also be needed.

Tuberculosis
Definition
Tuberculosis (TB) is a notifiable (in the UK) communicable disease caused by *Mycobacterium tuberculosis*. TB is found in the lungs (pulmonary) and in other parts of the body (extra-pulmonary), such as lymph nodes, CNS, bones and joints. TB is spread by respiratory droplets.

TB can affect a person of any age. It is more likely to affect immuno-compromised people and is a major global health problem.

Infection control is critical in minimising the spread of TB, and contact tracing is also important. Childhood immunisation is the most effective preventative measure against TB.

TB can be resistant to drugs, when it is known as multi-drug-resistant TB (MDR-TB).

Symptoms of TB include night sweats, fever and a productive cough. People with advanced TB may also have loss of appetite, weight loss and haemoptysis.

Diagnosis and investigations
History, examination and identification of causative organism.

Treatment
Treatment includes combinations of drugs (usually four) over six months. Adherence to these long-term drug regimens can be difficult for some patients and requires monitoring.

Nursing care
Nursing people with TB can span community and hospital care. Initially a patient is most likely to be nursed at home; only if their condition worsens will they be admitted to hospital. Nursing care at home primarily focuses on education about medication regimes and adherence to them and infection control. If the person is admitted to hospital, strict infection control procedures will be put in place until treatment is shown to be effective. Specialist TB nurses will advise about care and contact tracing. Prevention of TB is important, so health visitors, midwives, school nurses and practice nurses have a key role in ensuring that infants and children are immunised.

Ulcerative colitis
Definition
Ulcerative colitis (UC) is the most common form of inflammatory bowel disease (IBD). It is characterised by contiguous inflammation of the mucosa of the large intestine from the rectum upwards (colitis); widespread (but relatively superficial) ulceration may occur, resulting in chronic diarrhoea (often bloody) and malaise. Rectal bleeding, mucus and pus in stools and the urge to defecate without having any stools to pass (tenesmus) may also occur. Extra-intestinal problems such as iritis and skin lesions can develop.

UC usually starts in young adulthood. The cause is unknown, but some people may have a genetic predisposition to it.

Most people with UC experience acute episodes interspersed with periods when they are free from symptoms; in 10% of people UC is active all the time, while others (~10%) can experience long-term remission. A very small number of people will die from UC.

Diagnosis and investigations
History, clinical examination and scoping/imaging.

Treatment
UC is not curable, but is treatable with medication and/or surgery. Symptom management is important.

Nursing care
The routine nursing care of patients with UC focuses on health education and promotion and symptom control and management. These are particularly important aspects of care because many of the symptoms of UC are perceived as both embarrassing and isolating; minimising symptoms and these feelings will increase a person's sense of wellbeing. Medication will be prescribed by the GP/gastro-intestinal specialist and advice should be given about adherence and possible side effects. During acute exacerbations, some patients require hospitalisation for intravenous drug therapy, rehydration, parenteral nutrition, blood transfusion or surgery. Around 20–30% of people require surgery due to perforation, fistulae, abscesses or dilation with the potential for rupture. Regardless of the type of operation undertaken, patients and their family/carers will be anxious about the consequences of surgery (e.g. the formation of a stoma), so careful explanation will be needed – consultation with a stoma nurse specialist should be arranged if a stoma is likely to be formed. Depression may accompany UC.

Urethritis
Definition
Urethritis is inflammation of the urethra. It is the most common presentation of sexually transmitted infections in men, although irritants, inflammation and foreign bodies can also cause similar symptoms (e.g. pain on urination).

Diagnosis and investigations
History, examination and urinalysis and sample testing.

Treatment
Depends on cause.

Nursing care
Nursing care is primarily associated with sample taking for diagnostic testing and with health education and health promotion, such as advising the patient to avoid sexual intercourse until the infection has gone and reminding them that sexual partners will also need to be checked for infection.

Urinary calculi

Definition
Urinary calculi (stones) are solid concentrations of solutes in the urinary tract formed when they precipitate from the urine. Most calculi contain calcium oxylate. More men than women get urinary calculi.

Calculi present with haematuria and often very severe, sharp pain in the loin (acute renal colic) as the stones are moved along the ureter by peristalsis, supra-pubic pain, dysuria, urinary tract infections (UTIs) and urinary tract obstruction.

Acute or chronic renal failure can result from obstruction or consequent infection.

Diagnosis and investigation
History, clinical examination and investigations, including imaging of the calculi, blood tests for renal function, urinalysis, microscopy, culture and sensitivities to check for infection.

Treatment
Immediate management focuses on pain control (renal colic is extremely painful) and control of nausea with antiemetics. Increased fluid intake is recommended (3+ litres/day). Fluid balance needs regular assessment as diminishing urinary output or anuria suggests blockage to both kidneys; this is a medical emergency. Around 80% of calculi pass spontaneously without complication.

Most calculi are managed without surgery by extracorporeal shock wave lithotripsy (ESWL), percutaneous nephrostomy, ureteroscopy and lithotripsy to reduce the stones to smaller particles, or extraction of the calculi. Open surgery is rare (ureterolithotomy/ nephrolithotomy).

Nursing care
The nursing care of patients with obstruction of the urinary tract due to calculi focuses largely on pain control and careful observations for deterioration. Fluid balance is important in identifying early signs of diminishing urine output.

Urinary retention
Definition

The sudden inability to pass urine is termed acute urinary retention (AUR). The main causes include bladder cancer, benign prostatic hypertrophy (BPH), prostate cancer, prostatitis, prolapse (urinary, cystocoele or rectocoele), pelvic mass (fibroid, malignancy, ovarian cyst), calculi or faecal impaction.

AUR is very painful and is treated by emergency catheterisation. Once the immediate problem is solved, management of the underlying cause becomes the priority.

Nursing care

Nursing care will vary depending on the cause. In all cases careful attention should be paid to urinary output once the catheter is removed. Monitoring temperature for signs of infection is also important following catheterisation.

Recognising and responding to any sudden deterioration (e.g. reduction in urine, pain) in a patient's condition is vital. Complications include UTIs, renal failure and post-obstructive diuresis, which may lead to electrolyte imbalance with the resultant risk of arrhythmias.

Urinary tract infections
Definition
Urinary tract infections (UTIs) are very common. They are more common in women, which may be because women have a shorter urethra than men and most UTIs occur because bowel flora are introduced into the bladder via the urethra.

UTIs are commonly attributed to sexual intercourse, incomplete emptying of the bladder (e.g. neurogenic bladder in multiple sclerosis, spinal cord injury), urinary calculi, diabetes mellitus, structural abnormalities of the urinary tract and urethral catheters.

Symptoms include fever, pain, frequency, urgency and smelly urine.

Confusion often accompanies UTIs in older people – it may even be the only clue to these UTIs.

If symptoms are in the bladder, the inflammation caused by infection is called cystitis, which may be acute or chronic.

Inflammation caused by infection of the pelvis of the kidney is called pyelonephritis.

Diagnosis and investigations
History, examination and urinalysis with a dip stick for nitrites (suggesting gram-negative bacteria), protein, blood and leukocytes (inflammatory response); microscopy, culture and sensitivities of a clean catch of urine; renal tract imaging to look for underlying causes such as structural abnormalities.

Treatment
Treatment is with antibiotics. Usually oral therapy is sufficient, however acute pyelonephritis may require IV antibiotics. Persistent pyelonephritis may result in renal failure, requiring dialysis.

Increased fluid intake (3 litres/day) is recommended to flush the kidneys, prevent urinary stasis in the bladder and decrease bacterial replication.

Nursing care
The care of patients with urinary tract infections is largely focused on the GP, with treatment with oral antibiotics being the first course of action. In the main, people with UTIs require no specific nursing care. Sometimes, however, UTIs need more active management with intravenous antibiotics and this may require a short stay in hospital.

Vaginal discharge

Definition

Vaginal discharge is one of the most common symptoms that women seek advice about, either through their GP or practice nurses or from nurses working in family planning or sexual health clinics. There are several causes (not always related to sexually transmitted infections), including allergy, irritants such as a soap or bath oils, panty liners and spermicides.

There can also be a link between systemic disorders and vaginal discharge (e.g. diabetes predisposes a person to candida).

Diagnosis and investigations

History, examination and sample testing.

Treatment

Depends on the cause.

Nursing care

Nursing care is primarily associated with sample taking for diagnostic testing and with health education and health promotion, for example if appropriate advising about avoiding sexual intercourse until the infection has gone, and reminding the patient that sexual partners will also need to be checked for infection.

Valve disease
Definition
The heart valves can malfunction. Most commonly problems affect the aortic and mitral valves. Valve disease can be grouped into incompetence/regurgitation or stenosis.

Regurgitation is when the valve cannot close properly (i.e. is incompetent) and there is leakage behind it. This occurs commonly in the aortic and mitral valves. It is rare to find this in the tricuspid and pulmonary valves.

Stenosis is when the valves become stiffened and the cusps fuse together so that the opening of the valve is narrowed. This narrowing (stenosis) means that there is backflow through the valve into the heart chamber that expelled the blood. This may occur in the tricuspid, mitral or aortic valves. Stenosis may be a result of childhood rheumatic fever, particularly in the mitral valve, and age-related degeneration in the aortic valve. Congenital valve problems may also cause stenosis. Aortic stenosis and aortic regurgitation mean that the left ventricle has to work harder to pump blood out of the heart and this causes left ventricular (LV) hypertrophy. LV hypertrophy can eventually lead to myocardial dysfunction, arrhythmias and heart failure.

Mitral valve stenosis is almost entirely related to childhood rheumatic fever.

Regurgitation is commonly linked to age-related degeneration, infective endocarditis, inflammatory diseases such as systemic lupus erythematosus (SLE), rheumatoid arthritis and ankylosing spondylitis, and CHD. Mitral valve regurgitation can be caused by mitral valve stenosis or by stretching the valve ring when the left ventricle is dilated, as it is in left heart failure. Mitral valve disease can lead to heart failure.

Diagnosis and investigations
History, examination, echocardiogram, ECG and chest X-ray.

Treatment
Usually surgical replacement of the dysfunctional valve, either with a mechanical or a biological valve. Pharmacological control may be considered (e.g. diuretics, ACE inhibitors).

Nursing care
Nursing care centres on supporting the person and their family through surgical replacement of the valve or other invasive procedures, carefully monitoring their post-intervention condition and providing them with sound advice about their recovery and cardiac rehabilitation. Although people may present with symptoms of valve disease in primary care, their main interactions with nurses are likely to be in hospital.

Vascular disorders of the brain
Definition
There are several vascular disorders of the brain (e.g. stroke, subarachnoid haemorrhage, subdural haemorrhage and venous sinus thrombosis). Each has its own associated treatment and management.

The most common vascular disorder of the brain is *stroke*. Stroke – damage to the brain tissue due to either thrombosis or bleeding in the brain – can occur at any age, although it is most prevalent after the age of 65 years. Stroke is the largest cause of disability in the UK and the third largest cause of death after heart disease and cancer.

Stroke prevention is important, with raised blood pressure being one of the most easily modifiable risk factors. Practice nurses in particular have a central role to play in prevention.

Early recognition of stroke (or a transient ischaemic attack, TIA) can be lifesaving. The Act F.A.S.T campaign (www.nhs.uk/actfast) is an example of public health education and promotion related to early recognition and action. FAST is an abbreviation for:

- Face (face fallen to one side, inability to smile).
- Arms (inability to raise arms and keep them raised).
- Speech (slurring or inability to speak or understand).
- Time (call 999 immediately if you see any of the above).

Diagnosis and investigations
History, examination, brain imaging (CT and MRI), scan of carotid arteries and blood tests.

Treatment
Depends on cause and condition. Providing the best stroke care involves every member of the healthcare multi-disciplinary team, as well as colleagues working in social services and housing departments.

Nursing care
Nursing care in both hospital and the community (in people's homes, residential homes and nursing homes) will focus on the immediate management of stroke and rehabilitation.

Immediate acute stroke care will focus on minimising brain damage and resultant physical, cognitive and communication disabilities, providing appropriate and accurate information and reassurance to the patient and their family/carers, ensuring that the patient is nursed in a safe and comfortable environment (e.g. careful positioning in bed/ chair ensuring appropriate support of weakened limbs) and dealing with symptoms as they present (e.g. swallowing, speech and cognition difficulties as well as alterations to mobility and the ability to undertake usual activities of daily living).

Following stabilisation of the person's condition, nursing attention should re-focus to observations for deterioration due to for instance a second stroke, infection (pneumonia) or VTE, and to rehabilitation. Rehabilitation will involve working closely with physiotherapists, occupational therapists, speech and language therapists and the patient's family/carers.

People who have had strokes recover in different ways – some make a complete recovery, some have minimal residual disabilities, and some have severe disabilities and require ongoing complete care. People recover at a different pace, so individualised care is especially important.

Venous thromboembolism
Definition
Venous thromboembolism (VTE) is a blockage in the circulatory system (either a DVT or a PE). A *pulmonary embolism* (PE) is a blockage in the pulmonary arterial system. In this instance emboli can result from a blood clot emanating from a deep vein thrombosis (in the leg or pelvis) or fat from a fractured long bone or orthopaedic surgery, or amniotic fluid or air (e.g. from bronchial trauma) or a small piece of tumour. PE is a medical emergency.

Symptoms and signs can be varied and may include breathlessness, cough, haemoptysis (coughing up blood), pleuritic pain, dizziness and fainting, hypoxia (confusion, agitation) and circulatory collapse (hypotension, tachycardia and hypoxia).

Treatment will include oxygen administration; heparin initially, which will be changed to warfarin following diagnosis; thrombolysis if appropriate.

Risk factors include bed rest, immobility, surgery, lower limb problems (fracture, thrombophlebitis), malignancy, previous VTE (either DVT or PE), hypertension, chronic dialysis, obesity and COPD.

PE can present without many warning signs, so being constantly alert to its possibility is very important.

Deep vein thrombosis (DVT) is a blockage in the deep veins of the leg or pelvis. Signs and symptoms include pain/tenderness in the calf, calf swelling and redness and warmth in the calf. Prevention is important, including mobilisation and leg exercises if movement is restricted.

Diagnosis and investigations
History, examination, blood tests (D-dimer), ultrasound scan, venogram (DVT), chest X-ray (PE).

Treatment
Anticoagulation therapy and dealing with immediate problems.

Nursing care
If you are the first to notice the change in/deterioration of a patient's condition, get immediate help and stay with the patient in case there is further deterioration (e.g. requiring basic life support). Subsequent care will depend on the prescribed treatment, but will always involve accurate, frequent observations of vital signs and reporting these appropriately. Clear explanation is essential to patients and their families/carers after PE/DVT. Advice about reducing risks (e.g. avoiding immobility) and adhering to prescribed anticoagulant medication (and its monitoring) is important.

A PE/DVT is a frightening experience for all concerned, so appropriate information will help to reassure the patient and their family/carers.

References and Websites

References

Cairns D, Williams V, Victor C, Richards S, le May A, Martin W, & Oliver D (2013) The meaning and importance of dignified care: Findings from a survey of health and social care professionals. BMC Geriatrics. March 22;13:28.

Copeland G (2005) A Practical Handbook for Clinical Audit. London, NHS Clinical Governance Support Team.

Cullum N, Ciliska D, Haynes B, & Marks S (Eds) (2008) Evidence-based Nursing: An Introduction. Wiley-Blackwell, Oxford.

Dougherty L and Lister S (Eds) (2011) The Royal Marsden Hospital Manual of Clinical Nursing Procedures. Student Edition, 8th edn. Oxford, Wiley-Blackwell.

Francis R (2013) Final Report of the Independent Inquiry into Care. Provided by Mid-Staffordshire NHS Foundation Trust. London, Department of Health.

le May A and Gabbay J (2010) Evidence Based Practice in Practice. In: Lewith G, Cousins J and Walach H (eds) Clinical Research in Complementary Therapies. Elsevier, Edinburgh.

le May A (1999) Evidence Based Practice. Nursing Times Clinical Monograph No. 1. London, EMAP.

McCormack B, Dewar B, Wright J, Garbett R, Harvey G and Ballantine K (2006) A Realist Synthesis of Evidence Relating to Practice Development: Final Report to NHS Education for Scotland and NHS Quality Improvement Scotland. Londonderry, Ulster University. http://www.healthcareimprovements cotland.org/previous_resources/archived/pd_-_evidence_synthisis.aspx (accessed May 2016).

RCN (2008) Dignity: RCN Definition of Dignity. London, Royal College of Nursing. http://www.rcn.org. uk/professional-development/publications/pub-003298 (accessed May 2016).

Rigolosi E (2013) Management and Leadership in Nursing and Health Care, 3rd edn. New York, Springer.

Websites

Websites are a useful source of information for both healthcare professionals and the public. Information about almost every condition can be found on the web from patient associations and groups (e.g. Diabetes UK, Multiple Sclerosis Society, Alzheimer's Society) or organisations affiliated to health services (e.g. NICE, NHS Choices).

Reading and interpreting information from these various sites require nurses to triangulate or confirm findings from one site with another.

For service users it is important to have information that is written clearly and accessibly. The best places to find this are likely to be patient associations/groups and the Patient website.

Some examples for you to look at are:

Alzheimer's Society: www.alzheimers.org.uk
Diabetes UK: www.diabetes.org.uk
Multiple Sclerosis Society: www.mssociety.org.uk
NHS Choices: www.nhs.uk
NICE: www.nice.org.uk
A comprehensive set of patient information can be found at Patient: www.patient.info

Index